Personalized, Evolutionary, and Ecological Dermatology

Robert A. Norman
Editor

Personalized, Evolutionary, and Ecological Dermatology

Springer

Editor
Robert A. Norman
Professor, Department of Dermatology
Nova Southeastern Medical School
Ft. Lauderdale, FL
USA

ISBN 978-3-319-41086-9 ISBN 978-3-319-41088-3 (eBook)
DOI 10.1007/978-3-319-41088-3

Library of Congress Control Number: 2016949466

Printed on acid-free paper

This Springer imprint is published by Springer Nature
The registered company is Springer International Publishing AG Switzerland

Preface

As we move into the second decade of the twenty-first century, we in dermatology have exciting potential for new avenues of growth to add on to our valuable pattern recognition, diagnostic, and treatment skills.

The idea of personalized medicine has old roots. Maimonides, in the 1190s, advocated personalization of medical treatment and that every patient requires individual consideration. The doctor should not say, "This disease is similar to that other case"; rather, he should treat each patient independently according to the patient's natural constitution, individual psychology, and specific circumstances. The physician should try to cure not a disease but a diseased person. Maimonides cited Galen as saying that in deciding on a treatment the physician needs to observe seven things: "the nature of the sickness, the nature of the patient, his age, his habits, the nature of the town, the season of the year, and the constitution of the surrounding air." Now, in addition, we are able to add genomics and other tests to the mix [1–3].

Here is an overview of *Personalized, Evolutionary, and Ecological Dermatology*.

Personalized Dermatology

Personalized medicine (PM) and genomics is easily accessible based on the results of genomic testing from the results of a buccal swab test. PM is the customization of healthcare using molecular analysis to influence medical decisions, practices, and therapies for the individual patient [4].

New research data will be based on the use of evolutionary medicine and genomics to highlight how we can become more successful at finding the proper types of antibiotic or therapy and dosage for a particular disease or pathogen and build a competitive edge by prevention and risk management against invasive viruses, bacteria, or wrongly administered drugs [5, 6]. Certain fields of oncology and reproductive medicine have been utilizing genetic testing for many years. The current effectiveness of the recently created tests within dermatology will need to be measured to determine the need to create more tests.

What are the factors that provide acceptance or resistance to genetic testing? Key issues include the reliance on the accuracy of data, what action will need to be taken depending on the results, the importance of clear guidelines to improve therapy, the determination and timing of which vaccines will be the most effective for select populations, and concerns about government intervention and "snooping" and inappropriate use of acquired genetic data.

The biocultural investigation of personalized medicine will help us most effectively plan our future. The big question is: With limited resources and funds how can we get the biggest bang for our healthcare buck? First, we must establish the importance and efficacy of personalized medicine in dermatology and not simply an inevitable outcome of the genetic revolution. The basic economic climate of most HMOs is to spend as little money as possible to create the most profit for the stockholders. The political and economic climate is always a factor in the acceptance and implementation of any new technique. By redefining the insurance concept of "shared risk" to incorporate the newer concept of "individual risk factors" in personalized medicine in dermatology will require a major paradigm shift, but the use of genetic testing may improve the chance for biological and evolutionary success. To accomplish the inherent goals of personalized dermatology medicine (PDM), we will increasingly need to factor in the genetic importance of skin disorders as we progress in our profession.

Evolutionary Dermatology

As many authors have pointed out, we humans call ourselves "naked apes," yet we are covered with fine, unpigmented hairs that are actually ultrasensitive touch sensors. As the only mammals with such highly sensitive touch receptors all over our bodies, we require a brain as large as the human brain to process this constant sensory input from the skin.

If you could write a biography of the skin, what questions would you need to ask it? How was it treated during the earliest of times? What did people think of their skin? What diseases were prevalent and how did it affect society and the skin? What do people do differently now? What reassurance could the skin give us and what warnings would it reveal?

Could there be any protective utility in skin disease? Perhaps in psoriasis there is some hidden adaptive function that carries a genetic survival advantage. If the same genes that trigger psoriasis also control the intensity of bacteria invasion, then perhaps the combined 1–2 punch of an enhanced inflammatory response and thickened keratin layer allowed those with the psoriasis-predisposing genome to have survival advantage. The natural process of desquamation, where the skin rids itself of excess layers of keratin, is heightened in psoriasis and may provide a helpful response to discourage colonization of the skin's surface by undesirable microbes and maintain integrity of the skin by shedding faster than colonization can get traction.

Other protective roles for psoriasis can be seen with cutaneous tuberculosis, a disease that can bring on horrible facial destruction. Psoriasis first came to widespread attention in the medical community in the mid-nineteenth century, coincident with a high prevalence of cutaneous and systemic tuberculosis. As many researchers have reported, cases of patients with both skin diseases were essentially absent. Do psoriatic carriers protected from tuberculosis have a survival edge against the more disfiguring cutaneous TB? If the psoriasis carrier could be protected against TB, the predisposing psoriasis genotype could survive. Trials and research with the new biologic drugs that now blanket the medical journals and TV commercial airways have proven that psoriasis patients have inherent T-cell populations that indicate activated immune systems. And we know that one of the main contraindications for the use of any psoriasis-halting biologic is an active systemic TB infection.

Ecological Dermatology

As Wilson writes, "the skin is a surface that, like the earth, is subject to bouts of disruptive erosion and disordering decay. Those who study the skin, like those who study the earth, are keenly interested in morphology, distribution patterns and classificatory schemes." He adds that "some interesting similarities arise from comparing contemporaneous periods of thought about the terrestrial landscape with those marking the human landscape – the skin" [7]. We must examine our skin from a geo-historical perspective and factor in changes in terrain and the effect of ecological changes such as global warming.

I have always tended to look at the skin from a habitat and natural ecological perspective. When I am not working in my office seeing patients, I am often in the natural environment of Florida, hiking, kayaking, taking photos, and observing; these activities provide useful insights to evaluate skin lesions in an ecological way.

We know the common habitat of AKs and SCCs. Most live on the sun-exposed areas of the skin, particularly on the left arm of those who keep their arms out the window while driving, the face, the neck, the chest, the legs, and all the other areas of chronic sun exposure. In similar fashion, one is most likely to see a cypress tree with its stabilizing knees around the edge of a river or a ring-necked snake carrying its orange belly over moist woodlands.

All of this comes into perspective when discussing these maladies with our patients. The depth of penetration of the disease heightens our depth of understanding of the prognosis and potential treatment, from superficial BCCs to deep melanomas.

Dermatology skills include the practical evaluation of the topography and climate of the skin. Who hangs out with this particular character? What shows a mutualism? The sweaty intertriginous areas of the axillas and upper thighs are delightful arenas for fungi to frolic and breed. The rampant tinea versicolor infects up to 20 % of the population of Florida at any one time. As we understand more about what grows on us and how it all interacts, along with how the introduction of new antibiotics, biologics, and other therapies affect our skin's ecological balance, we will need a heightened sense of the importance and offerings of ecological dermatology.

What do we expect to find as we examine the terrain? We use ecological skills to help our patients all the time. The short timber of the cutaneous horn signals the observer to be cautious of the roots, in which the squamous cell layer may harbor a cancer. If a fire-like eruption occurs on the face, neck, and other areas exposed to sunlight, it may signal a photosensitivity reaction based on a current medication that permits the skin to be more vulnerable to the sun's rays. If we see atopic dermatitis on an itchy child, we also inquire about the rest of the common triad—allergy and asthma. If you notice a ring of warts on the finger of a 7-year-old, you look at the lips to see if hand-to-mouth behavior has resulted in an auto-inoculation. If upon inspection of the back of a nervous character, you note at the upper back and arms and other easier to reach areas multiple excoriations in different stages of healing in a forest of erratic depigmentation, with no involvement of the center of the back, we shift our diagnostic weight to the self-induced features of neurodermatitis.

I greatly respect other medical providers and their tools of diagnosis. Fields like radiology rely on representations and neurologists on scans and tests to hypothesize on inner maladies. A pathologist can be an enormous aid to our diagnoses, adding another set of eyes and a deeper view of a disease process caught in a moment in time. Perhaps no other field of medicine entertains the notion of visual, real-life pattern recognition more than dermatology. Dermatology lives in the observable and the palpable—the skin. Skin clinicians deal with life in the wild, not just the tamed and frozen tissue samples of removed body parts or representations on a screen.

The skin is an amazing, versatile organ and we discover more about its magic every day. We have good treatments and need to practice persistent prevention. The addition of personalized medicine with an evolutionary and ecological perspective, if used carefully and ethically, will help us to be even more successful. In addition to how best to utilize any new technology, we must keep in mind that our most compelling skills are showcased when we fully listen to our patients' narratives, understand their histories and problems, and provide the greatest help.

Ft. Lauderdale, FL Robert A. Norman, DO, MPH, MBA

References

1. Leibowitz JO. Maimonides on medical practice. Bull Hist Med. 1957;31(4):309–17.
2. Kottek SS. Maimonides: Rabbi, Philosopher and Physician, YEAR p. 338–39.
3. Maimonides, *Art of cure: extracts from galen* (ed and trans) Uriel S. Barzel, p. 108, cited in *On Asthma*, ed. and trans. G. Bos, p. 123.
4. Paving the Way for Personalized Medicine: FDA's Role in a New Era of Medical Product Development. Federal Drug Administration (FDA) WEBSITE?
5. Hamburg MA, Collins FS. The path to personalized medicine. N Engl J Med. 2010;363(4):301–4.
6. Mancinelli L, Cronin M, Sadée W. Pharmacogenomics. The promise of personalized medicine. AAPS PharmSci. 2000;2(1):E4.
7. Wilson P. Afterword: reading the skin, discerning the landscape: a geohistorical perspective of our human surface. In: Reinharz J, Siena KP, editors. A medical history of skin. Pickering and Chatto. 2013. p. 209–20.

Contents

Contributors

John Barksdale LMU-DCOM, OMS1, Nebraska, NE, USA

Daniel Butler, MD Harvard Dermatology Department, Massachusetts General Hospital, Boston, MA, USA

Jeff Collins, DO Advanced Dermatology and Cosmetic Surgery, Maitland, FL, USA

Robert R. Dunn, PhD Department of Applied Ecology and Keck Center for Behavioral Biology, North Carolina State University, Raleigh, NC, USA

Center for Macroecology, Evolution and Climate, Natural History Museum of Denmark, University of Copenhagen, Copenhagen, Denmark

Sara W. Faulks, BS Department of Dermatology, Wake Forest Baptist Medical Center, Winston-Salem, NC, USA

Steven R. Feldman, MD, PhD Department of Dermatology, Wake Forest Baptist Medical Center, Winston-Salem, NC, USA

Pam Kittipongdaja, DO Advanced Dermatology and Cosmetic Surgery, University of South Florida Morsani College of Medicine, Maitland, FL, USA

Michael Morgan, MD, PhD University of South Florida Morsani College of Medicine, Tampa, FL, USA

Dermatology and Cosmetic Surgery, Michigan State University College of Osteopathic Medicine, East Lansing, MI, USA

Lauren M. Murray, OMS IV Department of Dermatology, Nova Southeastern University, Tampa, FL, USA

Robert A. Norman, DO, MPH, MBA Professor, Department of Dermatology, Nova Southeastern Medical School, Ft. Lauderdale, FL, USA

Dermatology Healthcare, Tampa, FL, USA

Sharad P. Paul, MD, MPhil School of Medicine, University of Queensland, St Lucia, QLD, Australia

Director, Skin Surgery Clinic, Senior Lecturer, Faculty of Surgery, University of Auckland, Auckland, New Zealand

Adjunct Professor, Auckland University of Technology, Auckland, New Zealand

Asmi H. Sanghvi, BS, OMS IV Department of Dermatology and Cutaneous Surgery, University of South Florida, Tampa, FL, USA

Philip D. Shenefelt, MD Department of Dermatology and Cutaneous Surgery, University of South Florida, Tampa, FL, USA

Rebecca Thiede, MD, Department of Medicine, Santa Barbara Cottage Hospital, Boston, MA, USA

Marty Walsh, MS, OMS I Professor, Department of Dermatology, Nova Southeastern University, Tampa, FL, USA

Chapter 1
Genetic Testing and Personalized Medicine in Dermatology

Rebecca Thiede and Daniel Butler

Abstract The genetic basis of many dermatologic diseases is becoming increasingly apparent however its clinical application to an individual patient remains a challenge. This chapter aims to highlight the utility of genetic testing in the setting of screening, diagnosing and counseling patients. Gardner's syndrome, Peutz-Jeghers syndrome, Cowden syndrome, MEN Syndromes, Ataxia Telangiectasia, Wiskott-Aldrich syndrome, Familial Mediterranean Fever are highlighted as examples of diseases with cutaneous findings where genetic knowledge can help guide clinical care.

Keywords Gardner's • Peutz-Jeghers • Cowden • MEN • Ataxia Telangiectasia • Wiskott-Aldrich • Familial Mediterranean Fever

Introduction

The field of medical genetics helps elucidate the molecular basis of disease. In the last several decades this knowledge has also helped with the clinical management of patients and their loved ones. Genetic counseling, early testing strategies and therapeutic options are ways in which a knowledge of genetics has changed the practice of clinical medicine.

The link between dermatology and genetics is well known and clinically applied. However, because of the nuances of many genetic diseases, it can be daunting for any clinician to recognize, diagnose and manage some of the most complex conditions. This chapter aims to help clinicians connect the known genetics of a disease to beneficial clinical practice.

R. Thiede, MD
Department of Medicine, Santa Barbara Cottage Hospital, 55 Fruit Street, BH616, Boston, MA 02114, USA

D. Butler, MD (✉)
Harvard Dermatology Department, Massachusetts General Hospital, 55 Fruit St, BH616, Boston, MA 02114, USA
e-mail: danielbutlermd@gmail.com

R.A. Norman (ed.), *Personalized, Evolutionary, and Ecological Dermatology*, DOI 10.1007/978-3-319-41088-3_1

Gardner's Syndrome

Gardner's syndrome is a subset of familial adenomatous polyposis (FAP) with several prominent extraintestinal manifestations. Individuals inflicted with this syndrome develop hundreds to thousands of adenomatous colorectal polyps and have a 100 % lifetime risk for colorectal cancer, typically diagnosed by 40 years of age. Gastric, duodenal, periampullary, and small bowel polyps also can occur but have lower malignant potential. In this syndrome, there is also an increased risk for other tumors including desmoid, thyroid, hepatoblastoma, nasopharyngeal angiofibroma, pancreatic, and adrenal adenomas. Other extraintestinal findings include congenital hypertrophy of the retinal pigment epithelium (CHRPE), dental abnormalities, cutaneous lesions, osteomas, anemia, occult blood in stool, bowel obstruction, and weight loss [1].

The cutaneous lesions seen in this syndrome include epidermal cysts, fibromas, lipomas, and pilomatricomas [2, 3]. None of the cutaneous lesions have the potential to progress to malignancy, but they are important to identify since they can sometimes occur before the adenomatous polyps develop. Thus, early detection of the syndrome can prevent the development of inevitable colon cancer.

Genetics

Familial adenomatous polyposis, including Gardner's syndrome, is caused by a germline mutation of the APC gene on chromosome 5q21. It is an autosomal dominant mutation with close to 100 % penetrance.

Epidemiology

The overall incidence of FAP is 1 in 10,000 births.

Genetic Testing Recommendations [4]

Genetic testing of patients with suspected Gardner's syndrome should include APC gene mutation analysis.

Genetic testing should be offered to (1) first-degree relatives of affected individuals with an identified mutation at age 10–12 years or sooner in clinically suspected individuals and (2) individuals with a phenotype suggestive of Gardner's (or FAP) with >10 cumulative colorectal adenomas and/or suggestive extracolonic manifestations (duodenal/ampullary adenomas, desmoid tumors (abdominal > peripheral)), papillary thyroid cancer, congenital hypertrophy of the retinal pigment epithelium ((CHRPE), epidermal cysts, osteomas) with no known family history.

Recommendation with Known Mutation [4]

Individuals should be screened for colorectal cancer by annual colonoscopy starting at puberty or whenever there are suggestive symptoms such as chronic diarrhea, rectal bleeding, or abdominal pain [5–8]. (NCCN clinical practical guidelines)

Immediate colectomy if there is documented or suspected cancer or significant symptoms. Relative indication for colectomy with the presence of multiple adenomas >6 mm, a significant increase in adenoma number, and inability to adequately survey the colon because of multiple diminutive polyps.

Postsurgical surveillance should include yearly endoscopy of rectum or ileal pouch, and examination of an ileostomy every 2 years [9–16].

Screening for gastric and proximal small bowel tumors should be done using upper endoscopy including duodenoscopy starting at age 25–30 years [5].

Annual thyroid screening by ultrasound [17, 18]

Biannual screening should be offered until age 10 years with α -fetoprotein and ultrasounds due to increased risk of hepatoblastoma that most often occurs in the first 5 years of life [19].

Periodic abdominal CT imaging for desmoid tumors is not recommended but preoperative abdominal CT scan before colectomy may be considered if desmoids have been an issue in family members.

Peutz-Jeghers Syndrome

Peutz-Jeghers syndrome (PJS) is characterized by single or multiple hamartomas throughout the gastrointestinal tract, hyper-pigmented macules, and increased risk of carcinoma of both gastrointestinal and non-gastrointestinal organs. The slightly increased incidence of carcinoma includes but is not limited to the small bowel, colon, stomach, ovary, breast, cervix, testicle, and lung [20–24]. The overall cancer risk in these patients is up to 93 % with colon cancer being the highest risk [1].

The hyper-pigmented macules occur in up to 95 % of those inflicted with PJS and occur around the lips, oral mucosa, buccal mucosa, face, genitalia, soles of feet, and palmar surfaces [25]. This mucocutaneous pigmentation usually occurs within the first few years of life and may fade after puberty [26]. They can be differentiated from ephelides, or freckles, due to their location on the nostrils, mouth, and oral mucosa. It is important to differentiate the macules seen in PJS from benign ephelides due to the increased risk of carcinoma, bowel obstruction, and bowel infarction seen in patients with PJS [25, 27–29].

Genetics

Peutz-Jeghers syndrome is an autosomal dominant syndrome caused by a germline mutation in the tumor suppressor STK11/LKB1 gene, which encodes for a serine-threonine kinase on chromosome 19p13.3 [30]. A mutation in the STK11 gene results in penetrance of over 90 % by the age of 30 years [31].

Epidemiology

The incidence of PJS is estimated to be 1 in 8300 to 1 in 280,000 births [1].

Genetic Testing Recommendations [4]

Genetic testing should be offered to (1) individuals with a known family history of Peutz-Jeghers Syndrome and (2) individuals with perioral or buccal pigmentation and/or two or more histologically characteristic gastrointestinal hamartomatous polyp(s).

Recommendation with Known Mutation [4, 32]

Monitor for colon, stomach, small bowel, pancreas, breast, ovary, uterus, cervix, and testes cancers

Colonoscopy, esophagogastroduodenoscopy, and video capsule endoscopy for colon, stomach, and small bowel evaluation, respectively, starting at age 8 years. If polyps present, repeat every 3 years; if no polyps, repeat at age 18, then every 3 years, or earlier if symptoms occur [32].

Surveillance for pancreatic cancer should be with endoscopic ultrasound (EUS) and/or magnetic resonance imaging (MRI) of the pancreas annually starting at age 30 years, or 10 years younger than the earliest age of pancreatic cancer in the family.

Annual self-exam starting age 18, annual breast MRI, and/or mammogram starting at age 25.

Pelvic exam, pelvic or transvaginal ultrasound, and pap smear annually starting at age 25 years for ovarian, endometrial, and cervical cancer risk.

Testicular exam annually from birth to teenage years and ultrasound if abnormalities palpated or if feminization occurs since 10–20 % of benign Sertoli cell tumors become malignant [32].

Annual chest radiograph or computed tomography in smokers to evaluate for lung cancer. Provide education about symptoms and smoking cessation. No recommendation for surveillance in non-smokers [17].

Cowden Syndrome

Cowden syndrome, otherwise known as multiple hamartoma syndrome, is characterized by mucocutaneous lesions that are typically associated with underlying lesions of the gastrointestinal tract, thyroid, breast, and central nervous system. The hamartomas and neoplasms are of ectodermal, mesodermal, and/or endodermal origins [33, 34]. 70–80 % of patients are inflicted with polyps along the gastrointestinal tract, with the most common type being hamartomas, as the name of the disorder suggests, as well as hyperplastic polyps and adenomatous polyps [35].

Thyroid disease and breast disorders are common clinical findings in patients with Cowden Syndrome. Thyroid disease occurs in 75 % of patients with Cowden Syndrome, with a cumulative risk of thyroid cancer of 3–10 % [1, 17]. Breast lesions also occur in almost 75 % of patients with the most common manifestation being fibrocystic disease. Breast cancer is the most common malignancy of patients inflicted with Cowden syndrome with a cumulative risk of breast cancer being 25–50 % [1, 36–38]. Other common findings in these patients are macrocephaly, vascular malformations, and meningiomas.

Mucocutaneous lesions are considered diagnostic for patients with Cowden syndrome and occur in almost 90–100 % of patients [39]. Facial trichilemmomas, acral keratoses, and papillomatous papules of the oral mucosa are the pathognomonic cutaneous lesions seen [17]. It is important to identify these lesions as part of Cowden syndrome, because they develop prior to the internal and neoplastic manifestations of this syndrome [39].

Genetics

Cowden syndrome is an autosomal dominant disorder that results from a germline mutation of the PTEN tumor suppressor on chromosome 10q23.

Epidemiology

The estimated prevalence of Cowden syndrome is 1 in 200,000 [40–42]. It is suggested that the prevalence is actually greater due to Cowden syndrome features seen commonly in the general population [17, 40].

Genetic Testing Recommendations [4]

Genetic testing should be offered to (1) individuals with a family member with known PTEN mutation, (2) individuals with multiple gastrointestinal hamartomas or ganglioneuromas, (3) individuals with personal history of any of the following:

Bannayan–Riley–Ruvalcaba syndrome (BRRS)
Adult Lhermitte–Duclos disease
Autism spectrum disorder and macrocephaly
Two or more biopsy-proven trichilemmomas
Two or more major criteria (one must be macrocephaly)
Three major criteria, without macrocephaly
One major and ≥ three minor criteria
≥Four minor criteria

(4) individuals with one major or two minor criteria and a relative with a clinical diagnosis of Cowden Syndrome or BRRS for whom testing has not been performed with major and minor criteria as follows:

Major criteria:
- Breast cancer
- Endometrial cancer
- Follicular thyroid cancer
- Multiple gastrointestinal hamartomas or ganglioneuromas
- Macrocephaly (megalocephaly, ≥97th percentile)
- Macular pigmentation of glans penis
- Mucocutaneous lesions alone if:
  - One biopsy proven trichilemmoma, or
  - Multiple palmoplantar keratoses, or
  - Multifocal or extensive oral mucosal papillomatosis, or
  - Multiple cutaneous facial papules (often verrucous)

Minor criteria:
- Autism spectrum disorder
- Colon cancer
- Esophageal glycogenic acanthosis (≥3)
- Lipomas
- Mental retardation (i.e., IQ ≤75)
- Papillary or follicular variant of papillary thyroid cancer
- Thyroid structural lesions (e.g., adenoma, nodule(s), goiter)
- Renal cell carcinoma
- Single gastrointestinal hamartoma or ganglioneuroma
- Testicular lipomatosis
- Vascular anomalies (including multiple intracranial developmental venous anomalies)

Recommendation with Known Mutation [4]

Surveillance in affected or at-risk Cowden syndrome patients should include screening for colon, stomach, small bowel, thyroid, breast, uterine, kidney, and skin (melanoma) cancers

- Colonoscopy every 2 years starting at age 15 years [39]
- Esophagogastroduodenoscopy every 2–3 years starting at age 15 years [39]
- Thyroid exam annually and baseline ultrasound starting in adolescence [39]
- Monthly self-exam starting age 25, annual breast MRI, and/or mammogram
- starting at age 30–35 years for breast cancer screening [17]
- Annual endometrial sampling or vaginal ultrasound starting at 30–35 years for uterine cancer screening [17]
- Urine analysis with cytology and possible renal ultrasound for renal cancer starting at age 18 [43]
- Physical cutaneous examination annually at or before the age of 18 years for melanoma screening [43]

MEN Syndrome

Multiple endocrine neoplasia (MEN) syndromes are a heterogeneous group of disorders that are characterized by the occurrence of specific neoplasms. All MEN syndromes are autosomal dominantly inherited. Both MEN1 and MEN2 are discussed below.

MEN 1 Syndrome

MEN1 classically affects parathyroid glands, pancreatic islet cells, and the anterior pituitary. Parathyroid tumors, resulting in primary hyperparathyroidism, are the most common feature of MEN1 and occur in approximately 95 % of MEN1 patients [44–47]. Symptoms of hypercalcemia due to the excess parathyroid hormone can be evident in these patients and manifest with polyuria, polydipsia, constipation, kidney stones, and decreased bone density.

Pancreatic islet tumors are also classic and common occurrences in patients with MEN 1 syndrome. Pancreatic islet tumors, also referred to as pancreatic NET, consist of gastrinomas, insulinomas, glucagonomas, vasoactive intestinal polypeptidomas (VIPomas), and nonfunctioning pancreatic NET. At least one of these tumors occurs in approximately 40–70 % of MEN1 patients [46–51]. Symptoms depend on the type of pancreatic tumor such as recurring ulcers in patients with gastrinomas and chronic watery diarrhea with secondary dehydration in patients with VIPomas.

Lastly, the anterior pituitary tumors are the third type of tumor seen in MEN 1 patients. Anterior pituitary tumors include prolactinomas, somatotrophinomas, corticotrophinomas, and nonfunctioning adenomas. These tumors occur in approximately 30–40 % of patients [48, 51–54]. Like the pancreatic tumors, the symptoms from anterior pituitary tumors depend on their secretion. For instance, patients with prolactinomas may experience amenorrhea and gynecomastia.

In addition to the common manifestations of patients with MEN1, some patients may also develop adrenocortical tumors, lipomas, carcinoid tumors, facial angiofibromas, collagenomas, and meningiomas [48, 55].

Patients can commonly seek care from dermatologists for such things as facial angiofibromas, lipomas, and collagenomas with estimated penetrance of 85 %, 30 %, and 70 %, respectively [56].

Genetics

MEN1 is caused by a mutation in the gene, MEN1, on chromosome 11q13, which encodes a tumor suppressor protein, menin.

Epidemiology

MEN1 has an incidence of 0.25 % in the population [56]. This syndrome has a high degree of penetrance with >80 % of patients developing clinical manifestations and endocrine tumors by the fifth decade of life [44, 45, 48].

Genetic Testing Recommendations

Genetic testing should be offered to (1) individuals with clinical MEN1 with two or more primary MEN1 tumor types (parathyroid, pancreatic, or pituitary tumors), (2) individuals with suspicious MEN1 which includes recurrent hyperparathyroidism, gastinoma, or multiple pancreatic neuro-endrocrine tumors at any age OR multiple parathyroid adenomas occurring before 40 years of age and (3) individuals with atypical MEN1 syndrome (two or more MEN-1 associated tumors that are not part of the classical triad of parathyroid, pancreatic, and pituitary tumors), and (4) individuals with a first-degree family member with MEN1 [51].

Recommendation with Known Mutation [51]

- Annual assessment of biochemical tests for identification of MEN1 associated tumors
- Annual serum calcium and PTH concentration for parathyroid adenoma screening starting at 8 years of age [51, 57]
- Annual plasma gastrin starting at age 20 years for gastrinoma screening [51, 57]

- Annual fasting glucose and insulin concentration starting at age 5 years for insulinoma screening [51, 57]
- Annual serum glucagon, vasoactive intestinal polypeptide, pancreatic polypeptide, chromogranin-A for other pancreatic neuro-endocrine tumor screening starting by age 10 years [51, 57]
- Annual plasma prolactin and IGF-1 levels and pituitary MRI every 3–5 years for pituitary tumor screening
- CT or MRI of the chest every 1–2 years is recommended for detection of thymic and bronchopulmonary carcinoid tumors; urinary 5-hydroxyindoleacetic acid and chromogranin A is not helpful
- Gastroscopic examination (with biopsy) every 3 years in those with hypergastrinemia for detection of peptic ulcer disease and gastric carcinoid type II
- Abdominal imaging by CT or MRI annually for adrenal tumor and pancreatic neuroendocrine tumor screening
- Thoracic CT or MRI every 1–2 years for thymic and bronchial carcinoid screening [57]

MEN 2 Syndrome

MEN2 syndrome is characterized by early medullary thyroid carcinoma and includes two subtypes, MEN2A and MEN2B. Medullary thyroid cancer (MTC) is a calcitonin-secreting tumor. The risk of developing MTC in patients with MEN2 is high, with at least 70–95 % risk in patients with MEN2A and almost 100 % in MEN2B [58, 59]. MTC can present with dysphagia, hoarseness, diarrhea, and flushing.

Both MEN2A and 2B are also associated with pheochromocytoma, a neuroendocrine tumor of the medulla of the adrenal glands leading to secretion of high amount of catecholamines, epinephrine and noreprinephrine. Symptoms of pheochromocyoma include elevated blood pressure and pulse, orthostatic hypotension, palpitations, diaphoresis, headaches, and anxiety. Pheochromocytoma occurs in approximately 50 % of patients with MEN2 [60].

MEN2A is additionally associated with parathyroid hyperplasia leading to hyperparathyroidism and elevated calcium levels as seen in patients with MEN1. MEN2B, on the other hand, is associated with mucosal neuromas of the lip, tongue, and inner eyelids, marfanoid body habitus, ganglioneuromatosis of the gastrointestinal tract, and medullated corneal nerve fibers [61, 62].

Genetics

MEN2 is caused by a mutation in the RET gene on chromosome 10q11.2, which codes for a proto-oncogene tyrosine kinase receptor protein. The RET mutation results in constitutive activation of the receptor [63].

Epidemiology

MEN2 has an overall prevalence of 1 in 200,000 live births [64].

Genetic Testing Recommendations

Genetic testing should be offered to (1) individuals with clinically proven MEN 2 syndrome, (2) individuals with medullary thyroid cancer or pheochromocytoma and a family member with medullary thyroid cancer or pheochromocytoma, (3) individuals with sporadic MEN2-related tumors and young age (<35 years), multicentric tumors in one organ, and/or two different organs affected, and (4) individuals with first- or second-degree relatives with diagnosed MEN2 syndrome with RET mutation.

Recommendation with Known Mutation

- Prophylactic thyroidectomy regardless of calcitonin level [65]
- If thyroidectomy has not occurred, annual calcitonin levels [63]
- Annual serum metanephrine or 24-h urine catecholamines or metanephrine levels for pheochromocytoma screening starting between 8 and 20 years of age depending on the type of RET mutation [66]
- Patients should also be screened for pheochromocytoma prior to any surgery with treatment to identify need for adrenergic blockade administration [63]
- Annual serum calcium and PTH levels for individuals with MEN2A [67]

Ataxia Telangiectasia

Ataxia telangiectasia (AT) is a syndrome characterized by a spectrum of defects including neurodegeneration, immune dysfunction, radiosensitivity, oculocutaneous telangiectasias and cancer predisposition [68, 69]. The prominent neurological finding is cerebellar ataxia, which results in individuals being wheelchair bound typically before adolescent years. Progressive dysarthria, choreoathetosis, abnormal involuntary and voluntary saccades, and abnormal eye tracking are other common neurological findings [70–74]. immune dysfunction is a result of impaired humoral and cellular immunity, which leads to recurrent sinopulmonary infections with immunodeficiencies occurring in 60–80 % of individuals [1]. Individuals typically have decreased or absent IgA, IgE, and IgG2 [68]. The increased risk of cancer in AT is due to the genomic instability arising from this condition and includes an increased risk of leukemia, lymphoma, and breast cancer [68, 75–77].

The cutaneous lesion seen most often in patients with AT is oculocutaneous telangiectasias. Oculocutaneous telangiectasias appear around 3–5 years of age and occur primarily in the bulbar conjunctivae, over the surface of the ears and cheeks, in the corners of the eyes, on exposed parts of the neck, on the bridge of the nose, and in the flexor creases of the forearms [1]. Café-au-lait macules, hypopigmented macules, or melanocytic nevi may also be present in children inflicted with AT. It is important to look for signs of neurodegenerative dysfunction including ataxia, dysarthria, and periodic alternating nystagmus as well as identify if there is a history of recurrent sinopulmonary infections if an individual, typically child, presents with ocular and/or cutaneous telangiectasias, since these individuals are at risk for AT and have an increased risk of specific cancers.

Genetics

Ataxia telangiectasia is due to a mutation of the ATM gene, standing for ataxia-telangiectasia mutated, that is located on chromosome 11q22.3. The ATM gene is involved in detection of DNA damage and cell cycle progression by phosphorylating tumor suppressor protein p53 and other proteins in the presence of damage [78, 79]. It is an autosomal recessive disorder.

Epidemiology

The estimated incidence of AT is 1 in 20,000 to 1 in 100,000 births. As many as 1.4–2 % of Caucasians carry one defective AT gene [1, 80, 81].

Wiskott-Aldrich Syndrome

Wiskott-Aldrich syndrome (WAS) is an X-linked disorder that consists of a classic triad of severe immunodeficiency, microthrombocytopenia, and eczema [82]. The immunodeficiency in this disorder involves both T and B lymphocytes. Patients have decreased serum IgG, IgA, and IgM, increased IgE, and decreased T lymphocytes. Sinopulmonary infections are the most common infections seen in patients with WAS with acute otitis media being the most common manifestation and occurring in 65 % of cases [83]. Viral infections, fungal infections, and opportunistic infections such as *Pneumocystis jirovecii* are also seen in WAS [83].The microthrombocytopenia seen in WAS leads to several bleeding complications ranging from benign complications such as epistaxis, petechiae, and ecchymosis to more severe complications such as gastrointestinal and intracranial hemorrhage. Bleeding complications occur in >80 % of patients. Other complications that occur in WAS include an increased risk of both malignancies such as lymphoma and autoimmunity disorders such as inflammatory bowel disease, arthritis, vasculitis, cytopenias (typically autoimmune hemolytic anemia) and renal disease.

The classic dermatological manifestations include eczema, petechiae, and ecchymosis with the latter two occurring secondary to the microthrombocytopenia. The appearance of eczema in the first few months of life and the lack of response to eczema treatment, coupled with the hemorrhagic aspects of these lesions, should be considered manifestations for a clinical suspicion of WAS [84]. It is important to diagnosis early to initiate treatment and improve patient prognosis.

Genetics

Wiskott-Aldrich syndrome is caused by a mutation of the WAS gene located on the short arm of the X chromosome at Xp11.22-11.23. The WAS gene encodes for the WAS protein, which is involved in actin polymerization and associated coupling of receptor engagement, signaling events, and cytoskeletal rearrangement [82].

Epidemiology

The incidence is 1 in 250,000 to 1 in 1,000,000 live male births [83]. The estimated prevalence in the United States is 1.2 % of patients with identified primary immune defects [85].

Genetic Testing Recommendations

Flow cytometry analysis of WAS protein expression should be used as a first line screening tool for individuals suspected of having WAS, since it is a rapid and inexpensive screening tool.

Genetic testing should be offered to (1) individuals with first line relatives with Wiskott-Aldrich Syndrome, (2) individuals in which the diagnosis is suspected but flow cytometry of the WAS protein expression is normal, (3) at-risk couples seeking to avoid the birth of a child with WAS and want pre-implantation genetic testing [86, 87].

Recommendation with Known Mutation

- Intravenous IG (IVIG) at physiologic replacement doses [86]
- Prophylactic antiobiotic use in patients with recurrent bacterial sinopulmonary infections [86]

- Lifelong prophylactic penicillin after splenectomy [87]
- Immunization with conjugated and unconjugated vaccinations; avoidance of live viral and attenuated viral vaccinations [87]
- Prophylactic Bactrim to prevent *Pneumocystis jirovecii* [87]
- Immunomodulatory therapy and immunosuppressive agents for autoimmunity while maintaining careful evaluation for infection [87]
- Hematopoietic stem cell transplantation (HSCT) recommended in patients with HLA-identical sibling or a matched related or unrelated donor [86, 88–91]
- Splenectomy to improve and/or normalize platelet counts recommended if microthrombocytopenia severe and HCST is not being considered [86, 89]

Familial Mediterranean Fever

Familial Mediterranean Fever (FMF) is characterized by recurrent attacks of fever associated with serositis including peritonitis, synovitis, pleuritis, and pericarditis [92, 93]. Episodes are self-limited, typically last between 12 and 72 h, occur at irregular intervals ranging from one week to months to years, and begin within the first two decades of life [93]. Prodromal signs are common and include irritability, diarrhea, nausea, and vomiting [94]. Fevers can be the only symptom in patients, and the fever typically ranges from 38 to 40 °C. Besides fever, an abdominal episode is the most common manifestation, occurring in 95 % of patients. Other common clinical characteristics include arthritis, pleuritis, myalgia, and erysipelas-like erythema. The long-term complication of FMF is amyloid A amyloidosis.

The cutaneous lesion commonly seen in patients inflicted with FMF is erysipelas-like erythema. It is seen in 20.9 % of patients inflicted with this disorder [95]. The erythema occurs on the dorsal of the foot, ankle, and extensor surface of the leg. It is typically tender to palpation, resolves within 1–3 days, and can be associated with arthralgia [93, 96].

Genetics

Familial Mediterranean Fever is caused by a mutation in the MEFV gene located on chromosome 16p13.3, which encodes for a protein named marenostrin or pyrin [97, 98]. There are 14 sequence variants of MEFV that are commonly seen in FMF [99]. Most patients demonstrate an autosomal recessive pattern of inheritance [97, 98, 100].

Epidemiology

It has the highest prevalence in certain ethnicities such as Turks, Arabs, non-Ashkenazi Jews, and Armenians [101]. In these ethnic groups, prevalence ranges from 1 in 200 to 1 in 1,000 [102].

Genetic Testing Recommendations [99]

Genetic testing can include either targeted mutation analysis or sequence analysis of select exons [92]. FMF is considered a clinical diagnosis, which can only be supported but not necessarily excluded with genetic testing.

Genetic testing should be offered to (1) individuals with atypical cases when there are doubts about the clinical diagnosis (2) individuals with a family history of FMF with known disease-causing mutation [92, 99].

Recommendation with Known Mutation

- Colchicine to prevent and prevent FMF attacks and complications of FMF including renal amyloidoisis [92, 103]
- Annual physical exam including measurement of protein in urine [92]
- Consider IL1 inhibitors in colchicine-resistant patients [103]
- Consultation with auto-inflammatory disease specialist

Conclusion

Dermatologists are often responsible for diagnosing the clinical manifestations of these genetic conditions. While rare, it is essential that the field is aware of the appropriate clinical care in these cases and can help guide patients to the appropriate testing and management entities.

References

1. Ferris FFM. Ferri's clinical advisor 2015: 5 books in 1. 1st ed. Philadelphia: Elsevier; 2015.
2. Bisgaard ML, Bulow S. Familial adenomatous polyposis (FAP): genotype correlation to FAP phenotype with osteomas and sebaceous cysts. Am J Med Genet A. 2006;140(3):200–4.
3. Galiatsatos P, Foulkes WD. Familial adenomatous polyposis. Am J Gastroenterol. 2006;101(2): 385–98.
4. Syngal S, et al. ACG clinical guideline: genetic testing and management of hereditary gastrointestinal cancer syndromes. Am J Gastroenterol. 2015;110(2):223–62; quiz 263.
5. Vasen HF, et al. Guidelines for the clinical management of familial adenomatous polyposis (FAP). Gut. 2008;57(5):704–13.
6. Bjork JA, et al. Risk factors for rectal cancer morbidity and mortality in patients with familial adenomatous polyposis after colectomy and ileorectal anastomosis. Dis Colon Rectum. 2000;43(12):1719–25.
7. Bulow S. Results of national registration of familial adenomatous polyposis. Gut. 2003;52(5): 742–6.

8. Heiskanen I, Luostarinen T, Jarvinen HJ. Impact of screening examinations on survival in familial adenomatous polyposis. Scand J Gastroenterol. 2000;35(12):1284–7.
9. Parc YR, et al. Familial adenomatous polyposis: prevalence of adenomas in the ileal pouch after restorative proctocolectomy. Ann Surg. 2001;233(3):360–4.
10. Groves CJ, et al. Prevalence and morphology of pouch and ileal adenomas in familial adenomatous polyposis. Dis Colon Rectum. 2005;48(4):816–23.
11. Friederich P, et al. Risk of developing adenomas and carcinomas in the ileal pouch in patients with familial adenomatous polyposis. Clin Gastroenterol Hepatol. 2008;6(11):1237–42.
12. Tajika M, et al. Prevalence of adenomas and carcinomas in the ileal pouch after proctocolectomy in patients with familial adenomatous polyposis. J Gastrointest Surg. 2009;13(7): 1266–73.
13. Campos FG, et al. Rectal and pouch recurrences after surgical treatment for familial adenomatous polyposis. J Gastrointest Surg. 2009;13(1):129–36.
14. Ooi BS, et al. Anal transitional zone cancer after restorative proctocolectomy and ileoanal anastomosis in familial adenomatous polyposis: report of two cases. Dis Colon Rectum. 2003;46(10):1418–23; discussion 1422–3.
15. Tulchinsky H, et al. Extracolonic manifestations of familial adenomatous polyposis after proctocolectomy. Arch Surg. 2005;140(2):159–63; discussion 164.
16. Church J. Ileoanal pouch neoplasia in familial adenomatous polyposis: an underestimated threat. Dis Colon Rectum. 2005;48(9):1708–13.
17. NCCN clinical practice guidelines. 3 May 2015.
18. Herraiz M, et al. Prevalence of thyroid cancer in familial adenomatous polyposis syndrome and the role of screening ultrasound examinations. Clin Gastroenterol Hepatol. 2007;5(3): 367–73.
19. Giardiello FM, et al. Hepatoblastoma and APC gene mutation in familial adenomatous polyposis. Gut. 1996;39(6):867–9.
20. van Lier MG, et al. High cancer risk in Peutz-Jeghers syndrome: a systematic review and surveillance recommendations. Am J Gastroenterol. 2010;105(6):1258–64; author reply 1265.
21. Lim W, et al. Relative frequency and morphology of cancers in STK11 mutation carriers. Gastroenterology. 2004;126(7):1788–94.
22. van Lier MG, et al. High cancer risk and increased mortality in patients with Peutz-Jeghers syndrome. Gut. 2011;60(2):141–7.
23. Resta N, et al. Cancer risk associated with STK11/LKB1 germline mutations in Peutz-Jeghers syndrome patients: results of an Italian multicenter study. Dig Liver Dis. 2013;45(7): 606–11.
24. Giardiello FM, et al. Very high risk of cancer in familial Peutz-Jeghers syndrome. Gastroenterology. 2000;119(6):1447–53.
25. Utsunomiya J, et al. Peutz-Jeghers syndrome: its natural course and management. Johns Hopkins Med J. 1975;136(2):71–82.
26. Jewel Samadder N, Kory M, Jasperson W. In: Intestinal Polyposis Syndromes. Switzerland: Springer International Publishing; 2015.
27. Hinds R, et al. Complications of childhood Peutz-Jeghers syndrome: implications for pediatric screening. J Pediatr Gastroenterol Nutr. 2004;39(2):219–20.
28. van Lier MG, et al. High cumulative risk of intussusception in patients with Peutz-Jeghers syndrome: time to update surveillance guidelines? Am J Gastroenterol. 2011;106(5): 940–5.
29. Cunningham JD, et al. The role of laparoscopy in the management of intussusception in the Peutz-Jeghers syndrome: case report and review of the literature. Surg Laparosc Endosc. 1998;8(1):17–20.
30. Lebwohl M. Peutz-Jeghers syndrome. In: Treatment of skin disease comprehensive therapeutic strategies. Philadelphia: Elsevier; 2014.
31. Hernan I, et al. De novo germline mutation in the serine-threonine kinase STK11/LKB1 gene associated with Peutz-Jeghers syndrome. Clin Genet. 2004;66(1):58–62.

32. Beggs AD, et al. Peutz-Jeghers syndrome: a systematic review and recommendations for management. Gut. 2010;59(7):975–86.
33. Mallory SB. Cowden syndrome (multiple hamartoma syndrome). Dermatol Clin. 1995;13(1): 27–31.
34. Monga E, et al. Multiple hamartoma syndrome: clinicoradiological evaluation and histopathological correlation with brief review of literature. Indian J Dermatol. 2014;59(6):598–601.
35. Marra G, et al. Cowden's disease with extensive gastrointestinal polyposis. J Clin Gastroenterol. 1994;18(1):42–7.
36. Starink TM, et al. The Cowden syndrome: a clinical and genetic study in 21 patients. Clin Genet. 1986;29(3):222–33.
37. Brownstein MH, Wolf M, Bikowski JB. Cowden's disease: a cutaneous marker of breast cancer. Cancer. 1978;41(6):2393–8.
38. Eng C. Will the real Cowden syndrome please stand up: revised diagnostic criteria. J Med Genet. 2000;37(11):828–30.
39. Schreibman IR, et al. The hamartomatous polyposis syndromes: a clinical and molecular review. Am J Gastroenterol. 2005;100(2):476–90.
40. Nelen MR, et al. Novel PTEN mutations in patients with Cowden disease: absence of clear genotype-phenotype correlations. Eur J Hum Genet. 1999;7(3):267–73.
41. Melbarde-Gorkusa I, et al. Challenges in the management of a patient with Cowden syndrome: case report and literature review. Hered Cancer Clin Pract. 2012;10:5.
42. Hammami S, et al. Managing the risk of cancer in Cowden syndrome: a case report. J Med Case Rep. 2012;6:225.
43. Tan MH, et al. Lifetime cancer risks in individuals with germline PTEN mutations. Clin Cancer Res. 2012;18(2):400–7.
44. Thakker RV. Multiple endrocrine neoplasia type I. In: Jameson J, De Groot L, editor. Endocrinology. Philadelphia: Elseivier; 2010. p. 2719–41.
45. Machens A, et al. Age-related penetrance of endocrine tumours in multiple endocrine neoplasia type 1 (MEN1): a multicentre study of 258 gene carriers. Clin Endocrinol (Oxf). 2007;67(4):613–22.
46. Kann PH, et al. Natural course of small, asymptomatic neuroendocrine pancreatic tumours in multiple endocrine neoplasia type 1: an endoscopic ultrasound imaging study. Endocr Relat Cancer. 2006;13(4):1195–202.
47. Newey PJ, et al. Asymptomatic children with multiple endocrine neoplasia type 1 mutations may harbor nonfunctioning pancreatic neuroendocrine tumors. J Clin Endocrinol Metab. 2009;94(10):3640–6.
48. Brandi ML, et al. Guidelines for diagnosis and therapy of MEN type 1 and type 2. J Clin Endocrinol Metab. 2001;86(12):5658–71.
49. Thomas-Marques L, et al. Prospective endoscopic ultrasonographic evaluation of the frequency of nonfunctioning pancreaticoduodenal endocrine tumors in patients with multiple endocrine neoplasia type 1. Am J Gastroenterol. 2006;101(2):266–73.
50. Gibril F, et al. Prospective study of the natural history of gastrinoma in patients with MEN1: definition of an aggressive and a nonaggressive form. J Clin Endocrinol Metab. 2001;86(11):5282–93.
51. Thakker RV, et al. Clinical practice guidelines for multiple endocrine neoplasia type 1 (MEN1). J Clin Endocrinol Metab. 2012;97(9):2990–3011.
52. Trouillas J, et al. Pituitary tumors and hyperplasia in multiple endocrine neoplasia type 1 syndrome (MEN1): a case-control study in a series of 77 patients versus 2509 non-MEN1 patients. Am J Surg Pathol. 2008;32(4):534–43.
53. Verges B, et al. Pituitary disease in MEN type 1 (MEN1): data from the France-Belgium MEN1 multicenter study. J Clin Endocrinol Metab. 2002;87(2):457–65.
54. Sakurai A, et al. Multiple endocrine neoplasia type 1 in Japan: establishment and analysis of a multicentre database. Clin Endocrinol (Oxf). 2012;76(4):533–9.
55. Asgharian B, et al. Meningiomas may be a component tumor of multiple endocrine neoplasia type 1. Clin Cancer Res. 2004;10(3):869–80.

56. Degroot LJ, Jameson JL. 148 multiple endrocrine neoplasia type I. In: Endocrinology: adult and pediatric. Philadelphia: Saunders/Elsevier; 2010.
57. Marini F, Giusti F, Brandi ML. Genetic test in multiple endocrine neoplasia type 1 syndrome: an evolving story. World J Exp Med. 2015;5(2):124–9.
58. Howe JR, Norton JA, Wells Jr SA. Prevalence of pheochromocytoma and hyperparathyroidism in multiple endocrine neoplasia type 2A: results of long-term follow-up. Surgery. 1993;114(6):1070–7.
59. Eng C, et al. The relationship between specific RET proto-oncogene mutations and disease phenotype in multiple endocrine neoplasia type 2. International RET mutation consortium analysis. JAMA. 1996;276(19):1575–9.
60. Lairmore TC, et al. Management of pheochromocytomas in patients with multiple endocrine neoplasia type 2 syndromes. Ann Surg. 1993;217(6):595–601; discussion 601–3.
61. Wray CJ, et al. Failure to recognize multiple endocrine neoplasia 2B: more common than we think? Ann Surg Oncol. 2008;15(1):293–301.
62. Brauckhoff M, et al. Premonitory symptoms preceding metastatic medullary thyroid cancer in MEN 2B: An exploratory analysis. Surgery. 2008;144(6):1044–50; discussion 1050–3.
63. Lodish M. Multiple endocrine neoplasia type 2. Front Horm Res. 2013;41:16–29.
64. Moline J, Eng C. Multiple endocrine neoplasia type 2: an overview. Genet Med. 2011;13(9):755–64.
65. Skinner MA, et al. Prophylactic thyroidectomy in multiple endocrine neoplasia type 2A. N Engl J Med. 2005;353(11):1105–13.
66. Chen H, et al. The North American Neuroendocrine Tumor Society consensus guideline for the diagnosis and management of neuroendocrine tumors: pheochromocytoma, paraganglioma, and medullary thyroid cancer. Pancreas. 2010;39(6):775–83.
67. Kloos RT, et al. Medullary thyroid cancer: management guidelines of the American Thyroid Association. Thyroid. 2009;19(6):565–612.
68. McKinnon PJ. ATM and ataxia telangiectasia. EMBO Rep. 2004;5(8):772–6.
69. Woods CG, Taylor AM. Ataxia telangiectasia in the British Isles: the clinical and laboratory features of 70 affected individuals. Q J Med. 1992;82(298):169–79.
70. Crawford TO. Ataxia telangiectasia. Semin Pediatr Neurol. 1998;5(4):287–94.
71. Gatti RA, et al. The pathogenesis of ataxia-telangiectasia. Learning from a Rosetta Stone. Clin Rev Allergy Immunol. 2001;20(1):87–108.
72. Sedgwick RP, Boder E. Ataxia-Telangiectasia. In: Handbook of clinical neurology. Philadelphia: Elsevier Publishing; Vol. 60. 1991. p. 347–423.
73. Lewis RF, Lederman HM, Crawford TO. Ocular motor abnormalities in ataxia telangiectasia. Ann Neurol. 1999;46(3):287–95.
74. Baloh RW, Yee RD, Boder E. Eye movements in ataxia-telangiectasia. Neurology. 1978; 28(11):1099–104.
75. Gumy-Pause F, Wacker P, Sappino AP. ATM gene and lymphoid malignancies. Leukemia. 2004;18(2):238–42.
76. Angele S, et al. ATM haplotypes and cellular response to DNA damage: association with breast cancer risk and clinical radiosensitivity. Cancer Res. 2003;63(24):8717–25.
77. Thorstenson YR, et al. Contributions of ATM mutations to familial breast and ovarian cancer. Cancer Res. 2003;63(12):3325–33.
78. Ambrose M, Gatti RA. Pathogenesis of ataxia-telangiectasia: the next generation of ATM functions. Blood. 2013;121(20):4036–45.
79. Khanna KK, et al. ATM associates with and phosphorylates p53: mapping the region of interaction. Nat Genet. 1998;20(4):398–400.
80. Swift M, et al. The incidence and gene frequency of ataxia-telangiectasia in the United States. Am J Hum Genet. 1986;39(5):573–83.
81. Swift M, et al. Breast and other cancers in families with ataxia-telangiectasia. N Engl J Med. 1987;316(21):1289–94.
82. Massaad MJ, Ramesh N, Geha RS. Wiskott-Aldrich syndrome: a comprehensive review. Ann N Y Acad Sci. 2013;1285:26–43.

83. Sullivan KE, et al. A multiinstitutional survey of the Wiskott-Aldrich syndrome. J Pediatr. 1994;125(6 Pt 1):876–85.
84. Loyola Presa JG, et al. Cutaneous manifestations in patients with Wiskott-Aldrich syndrome submitted to haematopoietic stem cell transplantation. Arch Dis Child. 2013;98(4):304–7.
85. Modell V, et al. Global study of primary immunodeficiency diseases (PI)–diagnosis, treatment, and economic impact: an updated report from the Jeffrey Modell Foundation. Immunol Res. 2011;51(1):61–70.
86. Litzman J, et al. Intravenous immunoglobulin, splenectomy, and antibiotic prophylaxis in Wiskott-Aldrich syndrome. Arch Dis Child. 1996;75(5):436–9.
87. Buchbinder D, Nugent DJ, Fillipovich AH. Wiskott-Aldrich syndrome: diagnosis, current management, and emerging treatments. Appl Clin Genet. 2014;7:55–66.
88. Mahlaoui N, et al. Characteristics and outcome of early-onset, severe forms of Wiskott-Aldrich syndrome. Blood. 2013;121(9):1510–6.
89. Ozsahin H, et al. Long-term outcome following hematopoietic stem-cell transplantation in Wiskott-Aldrich syndrome: collaborative study of the European Society for Immunodeficiencies and European Group for Blood and Marrow Transplantation. Blood. 2008;111(1):439–45.
90. Antoine C, et al. Long-term survival and transplantation of haemopoietic stem cells for immunodeficiencies: report of the European experience 1968–99. Lancet. 2003;361(9357): 553–60.
91. Gungor T, et al. Reduced-intensity conditioning and HLA-matched haemopoietic stem-cell transplantation in patients with chronic granulomatous disease: a prospective multicentre study. Lancet. 2014;383(9915):436–48.
92. Shohat M, Halpern GJ. Familial Mediterranean fever–a review. Genet Med. 2011;13(6): 487–98.
93. Kucuk A, et al. Familial Mediterranean fever. Acta Medica (Hradec Kralove). 2014;57(3): 97–104.
94. Lidar M, et al. The prodrome: a prominent yet overlooked pre-attack manifestation of familial Mediterranean fever. J Rheumatol. 2006;33(6):1089–92.
95. Tunca M, et al. Familial Mediterranean fever (FMF) in Turkey: results of a nationwide multicenter study. Medicine (Baltimore). 2005;84(1):1–11.
96. El-Shanti H, Majeed HA, El-Khateeb M. Familial mediterranean fever in Arabs. Lancet. 2006;367(9515):1016–24.
97. A candidate gene for familial Mediterranean fever. Nat Genet. 1997;17(1):25–31.
98. Ancient missense mutations in a new member of the RoRet gene family are likely to cause familial Mediterranean fever. The International FMF Consortium. Cell. 1997;90(4): 797–807.
99. Giancane G, et al. Evidence-based recommendations for genetic diagnosis of familial Mediterranean fever. Ann Rheum Dis. 2015;74(4):635–41.
100. Stoffels M, et al. MEFV mutations affecting pyrin amino acid 577 cause autosomal dominant autoinflammatory disease. Ann Rheum Dis. 2014;73(2):455–61.
101. Ben-Chetrit E, Touitou I. Familial mediterranean Fever in the world. Arthritis Rheum. 2009;61(10):1447–53.
102. Onen F. Familial Mediterranean fever. Rheumatol Int. 2006;26(6):489–96.
103. Hentgen V, et al. Evidence-based recommendations for the practical management of Familial Mediterranean fever. Semin Arthritis Rheum. 2013;43(3):387–91.

Chapter 2
Genetic and Epigenetic Testing in Integrative Dermatology

Philip D. Shenefelt

Abstract The human genome consists of about 100,000 genes, of which approximately 20,000 code for structural peptides and proteins. Most of the remainder are control genes similar to off-on switches or other regulatory mechanisms. Epigenetics involves regulation of gene activation and deactivation through DNA methylation, alterations in histone structure, microRNA activity, and other factors. Genetic skin disorders, inflammatory and immune responses, and benign and malignant tumors all have genetic and epigenetic aspects. Understanding these genetic and epigenetic influences can assist in integrative management of common skin disorders as discussed in this chapter.

Keywords Genetics • Epigenetics • Integrative • Skin disorder • Methylation • microRNA

Introduction

Of the roughly 100,000 genes in the human genome, about 20,000 code for structural elements such a peptides and proteins [1]. Most of the remainder are control genes, off-on switches or other control processes [2]. They determine which genes in a given cell are turned on or off or otherwise regulated through DNA methylation/demethylation and alterations in histone structure. Noncoding RNA such as microRNA may also play a role [3]. These switches are affected by the external and internal environment. An environmental example for skin would be sun exposure with the effect of ultraviolet light on the cells. Advances in genetics and epigenetics are helping us to understand how skin cells are damaged, how skin neoplasia form and are dealt with by the body, and how skin inflammation is turned on and turned

---

P.D. Shenefelt, MD
Department of Dermatology and Cutaneous Surgery, University of South Florida, 12901 Bruce B. Downs Blvd, Tampa, FL 33612, USA
e-mail: pshenefe@health.usf.edu

R.A. Norman (ed.), *Personalized, Evolutionary, and Ecological Dermatology*,
DOI 10.1007/978-3-319-41088-3_2

off [4]. This new knowledge helps us to integrate genetic and epigenetic understandings of skin health and disease with diagnosis and treatment of skin disorders.

Skin and the nervous system develop side by side in the ectoderm of the fetus, with skin cells differentiating into keratinocytes and melanocytes and cells of skin appendage structures such as hair follicles, sweat glands, and nail matrix accompanied by fibroblasts from the mesoderm, tiny blood vessels, and nerve fibers. This highly complex process is regulated by cell type specific gene expression. Congenital and genetic skin conditions can manifest during this process. Examples include various types of congenital nevi and other congenital skin malformations. Genetic skin disorders such as incontinentia pigmenti, various disorders of keratinization, various basement membrane associated genetic disorders, and many others can be present at birth or can manifest later in development. Both genetic and epigenetic factors are involved in each of these processes. Information about many genodermatoses and their inheritance patterns is available in Spitz [5] and other texts.

Genetic testing can be performed on tissue obtained from lesional skin or normal skin with biopsy and with processing instructions as required by the laboratory. Interpreting results of the tests is usually reasonably straightforward for simple Mendelian autosomal dominant, autosomal recessive, and sex-linked genodermatoses. However, for many common skin conditions which have multifactorial inheritance and epigenetic aspects, genetic testing is not so simple and epigenetic testing even less so. These skin conditions and their polyfactoral genetics and epigenetics will be discussed in more detail below. Whether genetic repair will be feasible for any of these skin conditions is currently an open question.

Inflammatory and immune responses also differentiate within keratinocytes, Langerhans cells, B and T lymphocytes [6], macrophages, mast cells, and other participants in the inflammatory and immune processes. Again genetics and epigenetics is heavily involved in normal healthy skin as well as in inflammatory skin diseases such as psoriasis, atopic dermatitis, lupus erythematosus, various autoimmune blistering disorders, systemic sclerosis, and many others. Inflammatory and immune responses also occur in response to various bacterial, fungal, and viral infections and arthropod infestations of the skin.

Benign and malignant tumors of the skin also occur following patterns of genetics, genetic damage, and epigenetics. As an example of environmental influence, Parker et al. [7] demonstrated that nude mice exposed to the stress of smelling fox urine developed squamous cell carcinomas of the skin twice as rapidly when exposed to ultraviolet light as non-stressed mice. Common skin cancers such as basal cell carcinoma, squamous cell carcinoma, and melanoma have demonstrable genetic anomalies as well as epigenetic factors promoting their development.

Skin repair and healing as well as skin aging are also under genetic and epigenetic control as well as environmental influence. Ultraviolet light exposure, skin pigmentation, and cigarette smoking are all factors in skin aging in addition to the natural aging process.

Integrative dermatology involves selecting the best options for diagnosis and treatment of an individual patient. The diagnostic and treatment options are selected as appropriate from Western allopathic medicine, dietary and nutritional considerations, topical botanicals, herbal medicine, traditional Chinese medicine, ayurvedic medicine, hypnosis, psychosomatic hypnoanalysis, mindfulness, various types of energy medicine, and other creative choices [8]. Spiritual and religious dimensions may also be considered [9]. Skin and skin disorders and their treatments are evaluated on the physical, emotional, mental, cultural, mythic, spiritual, and energetic levels.

Genetics, Epigenetics, Testing, and Integrative Management of Common Skin Disorders

Acne

Based on twin studies of monozygous and dizygous twins, the heritable contribution to acne by additive genetic factors has been calculated to be 81 % [10]. The epigenetic processes involved in acnegenesis have yet to be elucidated. Tretinoin has been shown to suppress the genes involved in epithelial cornification and in lipid production [11]. Since *Propionibacterium acnes* is also involved in acnegenesis we are dealing not only with the human genome but with the bacterial genome and epigenetics as well. Integrative management of acne utilizes conventional allopathic treatments such as retinoids and antimicrobials, but adds appropriate dietary changes, botanicals, stress reduction methods, and other nonconventional methods [12]. Genetic testing for acne is primarily at the early research stage currently.

Aging Skin

Aging results in a time dependent decrease in skin function. Genetic and epigenetic factors play roles in this multifactorial process. A longitudinal genetic and epigenetic study of human skin fibroblast transcription, DNA methylation, and histone methylation has demonstrated an age-dependent decrease in expression of genes coding for proteins involved in translation and ribosomal function [13]. Conventional allopathic treatments include sun protection, topical retinoids, topical alpha-hydroxy acids, skin peels, laser treatments, microwave treatments, cosmetic surgeries, and other methods. Integrative approaches add when appropriate a healthy anti-inflammatory diet [14], emollients [15], and topical botanicals [16]. Stress reduction and practicing safe stress may also be beneficial. Genetic and epigenetic testing for aging skin is currently at the research stage.

Alopecia Areata

The usually patchy hair loss of alopecia areata results from T-cell mediated autoimmune reactions against anagen hair follicles. It occurs in about 2 % of the U.S. population. Genetic susceptibility linkages have been established on chromosomes 6, 10,

16, and 18 with those on chromosome 6 in the major histocompatibility region and on chromosome 16 near those associated with psoriasis [17]. There is a 55 % concordance in monozygous twins, a tenfold risk in first degree relatives, but no simple Mendelian inheritance, indicating a complex or multifactorial genetic susceptibility [17]. Abnormal epigenetic modifications have been noted in mononuclear cells from patients with alopecia areata [18] with genomic methylation increased compared with controls. Histone H3 acetylation was significantly increased and histone H3 lysine 4 methylation was significantly decreased in alopecia areata patients compared with controls. Conventional treatments include corticosteroids topically or intralesionally. Topical sensitization with dibutyl squaric acid is sometimes helpful. Integrative methods shown to be helpful include hypnosis [19]. Genetic and epigenetic testing for alopecia areata is currently at the research stage.

Atopic Dermatitis

Atopic dermatitis has a prevalence of up to 25 % in children and 2–3 % in adults. Seventy percent of atopic dermatitis patients have a positive family history. Twin studies indicate that genetic factors account for 82–84 % of the risk of developing atopic dermatitis, while environmental factors account for 16–18 % [20]. Filaggrin loss of function mutations on chromosome 1p21 are common in about 50 % of severe and 15 % of mild to moderate cases of atopic dermatitis. Another atopic dermatitis associated gene is the serine protease inhibitor Kazal type 5 (SPINK5) on chromosome 5q31. When defective it may be associated with accentuated Th2 responses, eosinophila, and elevated IgE levels. Epigenetic mechanisms contribute to phenotype plasticity and degree of severity. DNA methylation of the single cytosine 5' position adjacent to a guanine (CpG) on the filaggrin gene promotes loss of function filaggrin. The microRNA-155 also appears to be important in the pathogenesis of atopic dermatitis, and several other miRNAs are also upregulated and downregulated [20]. Conventional allopathic treatments for atopic dermatitis include topical corticosteroids, topical calcineurin inhibitors, and in severe cases systemic therapies such as oral corticosteroids, methotrexate, azathioprine, and others. Integrative treatments include topical soothing botanicals and oral kampo herbal mixtures [21]. Genetic and epigenetic testing for atopic dermatitis is currently primarily at the research stage. Delineation of various mutations and epigenetic conditions in atopic dermatitis has the potential to assist in tailoring care for individual patients based on these findings in the future.

Basal Cell Carcinoma

Basal cell carcinoma (BCC) is the most common skin cancer and is rarely metastatic but is locally invasive. About three quarters of the nonmelanoma skin cancers are of the BCC type. Genetic susceptibility to BCC occurs in autosomal dominant basal cell nevus syndrome with mutated PTCH tumor suppressor gene. This derepresses the G-protein coupled receptor Smoothened, permitting enhanced expression of the transcription factors Glis that drive basal cell proliferation and tumor growth. Patients with basal cell nevus syndrome develop dozens to hundreds of BCCs [22]. Chronic sun exposure can also result in a local mutation of the PTCH gene and subsequent BCC. Epigenetic methylation of the FHIT promoter has also been demonstrated in BCC [23]. Downregulation of the microRNA miR-203 has been noted in BCCs and likely also promotes proliferation [24]. Conventional allopathic treatments for BCC include excision, electrodessication and curettage, and Mohs micrographically controlled surgery. Thin superficial BCC may respond to the immunomodulator imiquimod. Advanced or metastatic BCC may respond to the Smoothened inhibitor vismodegib. Conventional prevention involves sun protection, and integrative prevention adds an anti-inflammatory diet. Genetic and epigenetic testing for BCC is currently at the research stage. Delineation of various BCC mutations and epigenetic conditions has the potential to assist in tailoring care for individual patients based on these findings in the future.

Lupus Erythematosus

Systemic lupus erythematosus (SLE) is a systemic autoimmune disease affecting women more often than men. Skin manifestations include a photosensitive malar rash, scarring discoid lesions, and a more diffuse maculopapular eruption. Autoantibodies are produced to nuclear molecules and other cellular antigens. The anti-nuclear antibody (ANA) test is positive in most patients. Genetic associations of SLE with major histocompatibility genes on chromosome 6 relate especially to genes for the complement components C2 and C4. Other associated genes code for opsonins and for complement receptors. Epigenetic changes in SLE include DNA methylation that alter T-cell reactivity, allowing development of autoreactivity that may also lead to B-cell ANA production. Two drugs that can induce lupus, procainamide and hydralazine, are both DNA methylation inhibitors [25]. Histone acetylation is increased in T-cells of SLE patients and upregulates some genes while downregulating others. MicroRNA miR-126 is upregulated and miR-142-3p and miR-142-5p are downregulated in CD4 T-lymphocytes of SLE patients [26]. Conventional treatments for SLE are usually primarily determined by the rheumatologist or nephrologist and may include oral corticosteroids, corticosteroid sparing agents, rituximab, and others. Sun protection is key for the skin lesions. Conventional topical corticosteroids may help to suppress the skin lesions. Integrative treatments of the skin can include *Aloe vera* as a mild anti-inflammatory and other topical herbal soothing lotions. Genetic and epigenetic testing for SLE is currently at the research stage.

Melanoma

Malignant melanoma of the skin is thought to arise from a series of genetic and epigenetic events. Sun exposure, especially strong intermittent sun exposure, plays a significant environmental role. Skin, hair, and eye pigmentation are genetically determined and also play a significant role in melanoma development [27]. Sporadic mutations occur with most acquired nevi having a BRAF mutation and most melanomas also having a BRAF mutation. Mutation of the NRAS gene is also a factor in melanoma development. While nevi do not tend to show chromosomal alterations, melanoma cells gain and lose chromosomal loci, with gain of several oncogenes and loss of several tumor suppressor genes such as P14, P15, P16, and PTEN. Family studies of melanoma have revealed three high penetrance germ line genes responsible for familial melanoma. The CDKN2A locus on chromosome 9p21 encodes the tumor suppressor gene p16 that regulates cell growth by arresting the cell cycle at G1, and also encodes for p14ARF that induces apoptosis and cell cycle arrest through p53. Two other rarer familial melanoma genes are CDK4 on chromosome 12q14 and BAP1 on chromosome 3p21 [28]. Epigenetic alterations in melanoma include DNA hypomethylation of some genes with activation, DNA hypermethylation of other genes with suppression, histone posttranslational modifications and chromatin remodeling, and some microRNAs downregulated and other microRNAs upregulated compared with normal melanocytes [28]. Aberrant CpG methylations of the TFAP2A gene has been shown to induce loss of TFAP2A expression in human metastatic melanoma [29]. The conventional treatments for melanoma include excision of the primary lesion with adequate margins, staging with or without lymphoscintigraphy, identification in metastatic melanoma of CKIT, BRAF, or NRAS mutations, and if appropriate in metastatic melanoma use of the BRAF inhibitor debrafenib or vemurafenib or the MEK inhibitor trametinib. Integrative treatment may add the anti-inflammatory diet. For metastatic melanoma, genetic testing for the V600E BRAF mutation is performed before considering use of vemurafenib, but epigenetic testing for melanoma is currently at the research stage.

Pemphigus

Pemphigus vulgaris is an autoimmune blistering disorder with IgG autoantibodies to extracellular cadherin adhesion molecules known as desmoglein 3 in the lower suprabasilar epidermis. The inflammation triggered by the autoantibodies results in loss of epidermal cell adhesion with blister formation. There is a genetic susceptibility to pemphigus vulgaris strongly associated with HLA-DR4 and HLA-DRw6. Epigenetic triggers may include viral infection and exposure to pesticides and sunlight, which are associated with epigenetic changes. For example, the Epstein-Barr virus increases DNA methylation of the E-cadherin gene [30]. Peripheral blood mononuclear cells from patients with pemphigus vulgaris have been shown to have increased DNA methylcytosine levels and lower histone acetylation and methylation levels than normal controls [31]. Conventional treatments for pemphigus vulgaris include oral corticosteroids, corticosteroid sparing agents such as azathioprine or mycophenolate mofetil, IVIG, rituximab, and other immunosuppressive agents. Integrative treatments include traditional Chinese medicine herb mixtures orally and topically. Genetic and epigenetic testing for pemphigus is currently at the research stage.

Psoriasis

Psoriasis is a chronic inflammatory T-cell mediated skin disease with multifactorial inheritance estimated at 66 % hereditary component and 34 % environment based on study of twins. Monozygous twins have higher concordance at 35 % in one study compared with 12 % in dizygous twins. There is a strong association between HLA-Cw6 and psoriasis. Epigenetic phenomena including DNA methylation, histone modification, and genetic regulation by microRNAs are regulatory factors present in psoriasis. Several genes in skin cells in psoriasis have hypomethylation permitting greater cell proliferation and one gene regulating apoptosis is hypermethlyated. Hypoacetylation of histone H4 is observed in peripheral blood mononuclear cells of psoriatic patients, and the degree of hypoacetylation correlates with the severity of the psoriasis. Specific microRNAs are increased and others are decreased in psoriasis. A small interfering RNA is also increased [32]. Conventional treatments include topical corticosteroids and calcipotriene, phototherapy, oral agents such as methotrexate, cyclosporine, and apremilast, and injectable agents such as biologics that act on factors such as TNF, IL-17, and IL-23. Integrative therapy may include fish oil, an anti-inflammatory diet, topical herbal extracts, and if indicated weight reduction. High hypnotizables may benefit from hypnosis to reduce psoriatic inflammation [33]. Genetic and epigenetic testing for psoriasis is currently at the research stage. Delineation of various mutations and epigenetic conditions for different types of psoriasis has the potential to assist in tailoring care for individual patients based on these findings in the future.

Squamous Cell Carcinoma

Squamous cell carcinoma (SCC) of the skin typically occurs on chronically sun exposed areas in relatively fair complected individuals. About one quarter of non-melanoma skin cancers are of the SCC type. Spontaneous mutations associated with SCC are in p53, RAS, NOTCH1, NOTCH2 and other genes, many not yet specified. Immunosuppression associated with organ transplantation is associated with higher risk of SCC. Familial cancer syndromes with increased risk of developing SCC include mutations in specific DNA repair genes. Examples include BLM on chromosome 15q26.1 in Blooms syndrome, PTEN in Cowden syndrome, FANCD1/BRAC2 in Fanconi anemia, TP53 on chromosome 17p13.1 in Li-Fraumeni syndrome, RECQL4 on chromosome 8q24.3 in Rothmund-Thompson syndrome, WRN on chromosome 8p12 in Werner's syndrome, and nucleotide excision repair genes in xeroderma pigmentosum [34]. Epigenetic changes due to DNA methylation have been noted in mouse skin cancer models [35]. Increases in some specific microRNAs and decreases in other specific miRNAs have been noted in SCC [24]. Conventional treatment for SCC is excision with adequate margins. Treatment of metastatic SCC is best referred to oncologists. Integrative treatment may add the anti-inflammatory diet. Sun protection is key for prevention. Genetic and epigenetic testing for SCC is currently at the research stage. Delineation of various mutations and epigenetic conditions of SCC has the potential to assist in tailoring care for individual patients based on these findings in the future.

Urticaria

Urticaria or hives are itchy skin welts where the individual lesion usually fades within 24 h. About 15–30 % of individuals will experience urticarial at some point in their lives. Acute urticarial resolves before 6 weeks. Chronic urticaria persisting for more than 6 weeks accounts for about 25 % of urticaria. Activated mast cells release histamine and other mediators of wheals. IgE is involved in allergic urticaria. Other urticarial triggers are autoimmune with IgG antibodies against the IgE receptor or against IgE, physical or pressure urticarial, cold urticaria, and cholinergic urticaria. Foods, food additives, drugs, especially aspirin, psychological factors, and viral infections are other triggers for urticaria [36]. Genetic mechanisms in urticaria have been associated with mast cell activation, the arachidonic acid pathway, and HLA class I and II alleles. Those with a history of atopy or elevated IgE level are at higher risk of urticaria [36]. To date, the epigenetics of urticaria has been little reported in the literature. Conventional treatments of urticaria include attempting to determine triggers and avoid them if possible, first line use of antihistamines to help suppress the urticaria, and second line use of corticosteroids, leukotriene antagonists, cyclosporine, dapsone, or omalizumab. Integrative treatments of urticaria include acupuncture, cupping, or a diet that avoids salicylates, preservatives, dyes, nuts, strawberries, fresh tomatoes, and seafood. Certain traditional Chinese medicine herbal combinations have also been efficacious [37]. For chronic urticaria, hypnosis with relaxation therapy has been reported effective [38]. Genetic and epigenetic testing for urticaria is currently at the research stage.

Vitiligo

Vitiligo is patchy loss of skin pigment associated with destruction of melanocytes by peripheral mononuclear cells. The prevalence is about 1 %. A genetic predisposition is indicated by a monozygous twin study that showed a concordance of 23 %, while for first degree relatives it is in the 5–7 % range. Epigenetic factors include increased DNA methylation of peripheral blood mononuclear cells in vitiligo patients and several microRNAs upregulated or downregulated in vitiligo patients [30]. Conventional allopathic treatments for vitiligo include topical corticosteroids and calcineurin inhibitors, and phototherapy with or without psoralens. Integrative treatments add herbal therapies including ayurvedic [39]. Genetic and epigenetic testing for vitiligo is currently at the research stage.

Warts

Warts are benign tumors induced by the human papilloma virus (HPV), a double stranded DNA virus of which there are over 120 types. The typical lifespan of an untreated wart is 5–15 years. Certain strains of genital HPV promote cervical cancer. Studies relating to HPV promotion of squamous cell carcinomas (SCC) of the skin are ongoing. The HPV virus has its own genome and its own epigenetics. Epidermodysplasia verruciformis is a rare genodermatosis, most commonly autosomal dominant, where mutations in transmembrane channel gene TMC6 or TMC8 create susceptibility to HPV with development of flat warts and increased risk of developing SCC [40]. Conventional treatments for warts may help to activate the body's immune response against the HPV that is required for resolution of the wart. Methods include freezing, painting or covering with acids, surgical removal or cautery, injecting anticancer agents or immune stimulating agents, application of immune stimulating agents, and others. Vaccines are available for prevention of oncogenic genital warts. Integrative treatments for warts include suggestion and hypnosis [41]. For refractory warts psychosomatic hypnoanalysis has often proved effective [42]. Genetic testing for wart type is currently available and is useful for determining whether the wart type has oncogenic potential. This is especially important for genital warts. Epigenetic testing for warts is currently at the research stage.

Conclusions

Research is just beginning to scratch the surface of genetics and epigenetics as it relates to skin and skin disorders. Only some of the more common skin disorders have been discussed here. Combining the insights and potential new diagnosis and treatment options provided by understanding the genetics and epigenetics of specific skin disorders with conventional and integrative treatments offers the individual patient the best that is currently available in diagnosis and treatment. With further advances in knowledge about genetics and especially about epigenetics, our better understanding of how skin disorders occur and how treatments work will continue to improve choices and outcomes for patients. Genetic and epigenetic testing for these conditions will become more routine in clinical practice, permitting a better knowledge based process of diagnosis and selecting appropriate treatments.

References

1. International Human Genome Sequencing Consortium. Finishing the euchromatic sequence of the human genome. Nature. 2004;431(7011):931–45.
2. Pennisi E. ENCODE project writes Eulogy for junk DNA. Science. 2012;337(6099):1159–60.
3. Jennin M. Various applications of microRNAs in skin diseases. J Dermatol Sci. 2014;74(1):3–8.
4. Lu Q, Chang CC, Richardson BC, editors. Epigenetics and dermatology. Amsterdam: Academic; 2015.
5. Spitz JL. Genodermatoses: a clinical guide to genetic skin disorders. 2nd ed. Philadelphia: Lippincott Williams & Wilkins; 2004.
6. Shih H-Y, Sciume G, Poholek AC, Vahedi G, Hirahara K, Villarino AV, et al. Transcriptional and epigenetic networks of helper T and innate lymphoid cells. Immunol Rev. 2014;261:23–49.
7. Parker JL, Klein SL, McClintock MK, Morison WL, Ye X, Conti CJ, et al. Chronic stress accelerates ultraviolet-induced cutaneous carcinogenesis. J Am Acad Dermatol. 2004;51(6):919–22.
8. Norman RA, Shenefelt PD, Rupani RN, editors. Integrative dermatology. New York: Oxford University Press; 2014.
9. Shenefelt PD, Shenefelt DA. Spiritual and religious aspects of skin and skin disorders. Psychol Res Behav Manag. 2014;7:201–12.
10. Bataille V, Lens M, Spector TD. The use of the twin model to investigate the genetics and epigenetics of skin diseases with genomic, transcriptomic and methylation data. J Euro Acad Dermatol Venerol. 2012;26:1067–73.
11. Lee DD, Stojadinovic O, Krzyzanowska A, Vouthounis C, Blumenberg M, Tomic-Canic M. Retinoid-responsive transcriptional changes in epidermal keratinocytes. J Cell Physiol. 2009;220(2):427–39.
12. Bowe WP, Glick JB. Integrative management of acne. In: Norman RA, Shenefelt PD, Rupani RN, editors. Integrative dermatology. New York: Oxford University Press; 2014. p. 223–41.
13. Jung M, Jin S-G, Zhang X, Xiong W, Gogoshin G, Rodin AS, Pfeifer GP. Longitudinal epigenetic and gene expression profiles analyzed by three-component analysis reveal down-regulation of genes involved in protein translation in human aging. Nucleic Acids Res. 2015;1. doi:10.1093/nar/gkv473.
14. Jacknin J. Nutrition and supplements for healthy skin. In: Norman RA, Shenefelt PD, Rupani RN, editors. Integrative dermatology. New York: Oxford University Press; 2014. p. 19–40.
15. Burris K, Hui AM, Akingboye A. Skin-influencing factors in daily life. In: Norman RA, Shenefelt PD, Rupani RN, editors. Integrative dermatology. New York: Oxford University Press; 2014. p. 50–64.
16. Hui AM, Siegel DM. Topical botanicals and the skin. In: Norman RA, Shenefelt PD, Rupani RN, editors. Integrative dermatology. New York: Oxford University Press; 2014. p. 223–41.
17. Martinez-Mir A, Zlotogorski A, Gordon D, Petukhova L, Mo J, Gilliam TC, et al. Genomewide scan for linkage reveals evidence of several susceptibility loci for alopecia areata. Am J Hum Genet. 2007;80(2):316–28.
18. Zhao M, Liang G, Wu X, Wang S, Zhang P, Su Y, et al. Abnormal epigenetic modifications in peripheral blood mononuclear cells from patients with alopecia areata. Br J Dermatol. 2012;166(2):226–73.
19. Willemsen R, Vanderlinden J, Deconinck A, Roseeuw D. Hypnotherapeutic management of alopecia areata. J Am Acad Dermatol. 2006;55(2):233–7.
20. Poliak N, Chang C. Epigenetics of allergic and inflammatory skin diseases. In: Lu Q, Chang CC, Richardson BC, editors. Epigenetics and dermatology. Amsterdam: Academic; 2015. p. 275.
21. Yamashita H, Tanaka H, Inagaki N. Treatment of the chronic itch of atopic dermatitis using standard drugs and kampo medicines. Biol Pharm Bull. 2013;36(8):1253–7.

22. Athar M, Li C, Kim AL, Spiegelman VS, Bickers DR. Sonic hedgehog signaling in Basal cell nevus syndrome. Cancer Res. 2014;74(18):4967–75.
23. Goldberg M, Rummelt C, Laerm A, Helmbold P, Holbach LM, Ballhausen WG. Epigenetic silencing contributes to frequent loss of the fragile histidine triad tumour suppressor in basal cell carcinomas. Br J Dermatol. 2006;155:1154–8.
24. Lovendorf MB, Skov L. MicroRNAs in skin diseases. In: Lu Q, Chang CC, Richardson BC, editors. Epigenetics and dermatology. Amsterdam: Academic; 2015. p. 177–205.
25. Strickland FM, Richardson BC. Epigenetics in human autoimmunity. Autoimmunity. 2008;41(4):278–86.
26. Richardson BC. Systemic lupus erythematosis. In: Lu Q, Chang CC, Richardson BC, editors. Epigenetics and dermatology. Amsterdam: Academic; 2015.
27. Greenberg ES, Chong KK, Huynh KT, Tanaka R, Hoon DSB. Epigenetic biomarkers in skin cancer. Cancer Lett. 2014;342(2):170–7.
28. Charlet J, Liang G. Epigenetics of melanoma. In: Lu Q, Chang CC, Richardson BC, editors. Epigenetics and dermatology. Amsterdam: Academic; 2015.
29. Hallberg AR, Vorrink SU, Hudachek DR, Cramer-Morales K, Milhem MM, Cornell RA, et al. Aberrant CpG methylation of the TFAP2A gene constitutes a mechanism for loss of TFAP2A expression in human metastatic melanoma. Epigenetics. 2014;9(12):1641–7.
30. Zhao M, Wu R, Lu Q. Epigenetics and other autoimmune skin diseases. In: Lu Q, Chang CC, Richardson BC, editors. Epigenetics and dermatology. Amsterdam: Academic; 2015. p. 307–26.
31. Zhao M, Huang W, Zang Q, Gao F, Wang L, Zhang G, et al. Abberant epigenetic modifications in peripheral blood mononuclear cells from patients with pemphigus vulgaris. Br J Dermatol. 2012;167(3):523–31.
32. Trowbridge RM, Pittlekow MR. Epigenetics in the pathogenesis and pathophysiology of psoriasis vulgaris. J Drugs Dermatol. 2014;13(2):111–8.
33. Denby K, Duffy N, Norman RA, Blackcloud P, Tausk F. Integrative management of psoriasis. In: Norman RA, Shenefelt PD, Rupani RN, editors. Integrative dermatology. New York: Oxford University Press; 2014. p. 373–89.
34. Ng Y-Z, Dayal JHS, South AP. Genetic predisposition to cutaneous squamous cell carcinoma. In: La Porta CAM, editor. Skin cancers – risk factors, prevention and therapy. Published: November 14, 2011, open access, INTECH. doi:10.5772/26714, ISBN 978-953-307-722-2.
35. Yang AY, Lee JH, Shu L, Zhang C, Su ZY, Lu Y, et al. Genome-wide analysis of DNA methylation in UVB- and DMBA/TPA-induced mouse skin cancer models. Life Sci. 2014;113(1–2):45–54.
36. Losol P, Yoo H-S, Park H-S. Molecular genetic mechanisms of chronic urticaria. Allergy Asthma Immunol Res. 2014;6(1):13–21.
37. Wilmer EN, Lee KC, Lio PA. Integrative management of urticaria. In: Norman RA, Shenefelt PD, Rupani RN, editors. Integrative dermatology. New York: Oxford University Press; 2014.
38. Shenefelt PD. Hypnosis, hypnoanalysis, and mindfulness meditation in dermatology. In: Norman RA, Shenefelt PD, Rupani RN, editors. Integrative dermatology. New York: Oxford University Press; 2014.
39. Madan R, Asrani F. Integrative management of Vitiligo. In: Norman RA, Shenefelt PD, Rupani RN, editors. Integrative dermatology. New York: Oxford University Press; 2014.
40. Burger B, Itin PH. Epidermodysplasia verruciformis. Curr Probl Dermatol. 2014;45:123–31.
41. Shenefelt PD. Integrative management of veruccae (warts). In: Norman RA, Shenefelt PD, Rupani RN, editors. Integrative dermatology. New York: Oxford University Press; 2014. p. 452–69.
42. Ewin DM. Hypnotherapy for warts (verruca vulgaris), 41 consecutive cases with 33 cures. Am J Clin Hypn. 1992;35(1):1–10.

Chapter 3
Forensic Dermatology

Robert A. Norman and Marty Walsh

Abstract Forensic dermatology is the field of science that refers to the examination of the body's largest organ, the skin, hair and nails, in order to search for a cause of injury, death, or disease. While dermatologists can use forensics on live patients, medical examiners will use dermatological forensics on the deceased in order to aid in police and medical investigations. The techniques that aid dermatologists and examiners can be beneficial in cases of abuse, bioterrorism, identity, and infectious diseases. A newer component to the field of forensics and dermatology is using the communities of bacteria and other organisms that reside on the skin, or the human skin microbiome.

Keywords Dermatology • Forensics • Microbiome • Medical examiners • Forensic dermatology • Short Tandem Repeat Analysis • DNA • Fingerprints • Sexual assault

Forensic dermatology is the field of science that refers to the examination of the body's largest organ, the skin, hair and nails, in order to search for a cause of injury, death, or disease. While dermatologists can use forensics on live patients, medical examiners will use dermatological forensics on the deceased in order to aid in police and medical investigations. The techniques that aid dermatologists and examiners can be beneficial in cases of abuse, bioterrorism, identity, and infectious diseases. A newer component to the field of forensics and dermatology is using the communities of bacteria and other organisms that reside on the skin, or the human skin microbiome. While there are commonalities in the organisms that thrive on the human skin, there are also differences between individuals. These differences in the systemic and dermatological microbiomes and the microbial DNA can be used as secondary DNA fingerprints in the criminal justice system. The bacterial DNA in the

R.A. Norman, DO, MPH, MBA (✉)
Dermatology Healthcare, 8002 Gunn Highway, Tampa, FL 33626, USA

Professor, Department of Dermatology, Nova Southeastern Medical School, Ft. Lauderdale, FL, USA
e-mail: skindrrob@aol.com

M. Walsh
LECOM Bradenton, OMS1, Tampa, FL, USA

R.A. Norman (ed.), *Personalized, Evolutionary, and Ecological Dermatology*,
DOI 10.1007/978-3-319-41088-3_3

microbiome can be left behind in systemic fluids like blood and gastroenterological excretions, dermatoglyphs, and tissue. Since bacteria contain their own DNA, this is a new form of criminal identification that is not restricted to only a criminal's personal DNA.

Forensic Science

The word "forensics" is derived from the Latin word "forensic" meaning "in open court, public" and is closely related to the word "forum" [1]. The modern definition includes "the application of scientific methods and techniques to the investigation of crime". Multitudinous areas of concern are used for consulting in the field of forensics like psychiatry, toxicology, zoology, and others. However, dermatology is an essential part of the medical examiners toolkit as dermatological changes can prove how a subject lived, died, and who they are.

Forensic Methodology

Forensic science relies on a technique called Short Tandem Repeat Analysis, which focuses on the Short Tandem Repeats, or STRs found in human base pairs of the DNA. Each repeat is roughly 2–6 base pairs in length and repeat themselves throughout the DNA, usually without consequences in mutated phenotype [2]. They serve as appropriate DNA markers in forensics because they can be created in mass amounts in a technique known as Polymerase Chain Reactions, even when DNA content is low or amalgamated in a sample. Also, STRs are unique to each individual person as half of human chromosomes are derived from the mother's ovum, and the other from the father's sperm, so they become perfect markers for one select individual. This same technique is used in differentiating bacteria and their DNA in a sample.

Patient and Victim Identity

Identity of a patient or deceased person is a very useful asset in aiding a criminal or medical investigation. Not only does it solidify a missing person's whereabouts, but also can also improve knowledge of targets and people involved in homicides, terrorism, and abuse. Fingerprinting is one of the most useful scientific tools because the different ridges known as whorls, arches, and loops of a fingerprint are unique to every individual [3]. Fingerprints are such important assets in forensic science because the statistics of two people sharing the same design on their fingertips is 1 in 64 billion [4]. Fingerprints are caused by ridges and recesses on the ventral

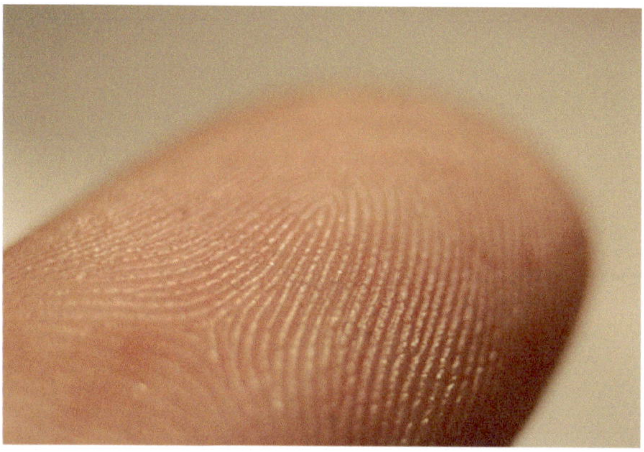

Fig. 3.1 Ventral surface of the index finger on a human male (From Wikipedia Commons: Schnell F. (September 28 2010). Fingertips Macro. Retrieved August 15, 2015. https://commons.wikimedia.org/wiki/File:Fingertips_macro.jpg. Licensed under the Creative Commons Attribution 2.0 Generic license)

surfaces of the upper and lower digits of the extremities, but the most commonly used for identification are the ventral surfaces of the upper digits (Fig. 3.1). The palmar and plantar surfaces of the extremities can be used as well for identification in cases where there is epidermal loss or fingerprints are not available. A dermatoglyph, or fingerprint, is left behind typically by any substance an individual touches and leaves behind on an object or another individual. If an individual doesn't touch another substance like blood, water, or paint, there are eccrine sweat glands that can leave behind the triglycerides, sebum, and chloride content that compose a latent fingerprint [5].

Approximately 60 % percent of the fingerprint is created by loops, which are lines that curve and retreat to the origin, whorls, which are concentric circles like that of a target on a shooting range (35 %), and arches, which are peaked lines that can be smooth or sharp (5 %) (Fig. 3.2) [3].

A problem in forensics for this type of identification is people who are born without or do not have fingerprints. A Swiss woman and a portion of her family members were born without fingerprints in a condition called adermatoglyphia. Her genotype was mapped and discovered she had a point mutation in the SMARCAD1 gene located in the chromosome 4q22, which caused her to be born without the loops, whorls, and arches in her digits that are associated with fingerprints (Fig. 3.3) [6].

There are other cases that result in adermatoglyphia such as the disease dermatopathia pigmentosa reticularis, Naegeli syndrome, and manual removal of one's fingerprints which is a temporary but painful technique [7]. Abnormalities of dermatoglyphs can also be found in those born with chromosomal and genetic abnormalities. These individuals include clinical syndromes like Klinefelter's syndrome with an XXY chromosome, Patau syndrome in Trisomy 13, and Down's Syndrome in Trisomy 21 [8, 9].

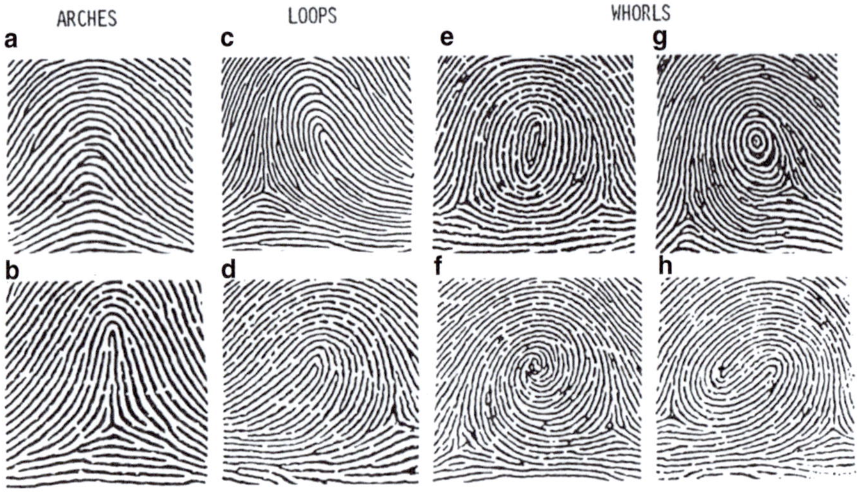

Fig. 3.2 Arches, loops, and whorls that are present in normal fingertips. (**a**) simple arch, (**b**) sbarp arch, (**c**) left loop, (**d**) right loop, (**e**) oval whorl, (**f**) spiral whorl, (**g**) round whorl, and (**h**) double loop (With permission from Coren [25]. © Springer)

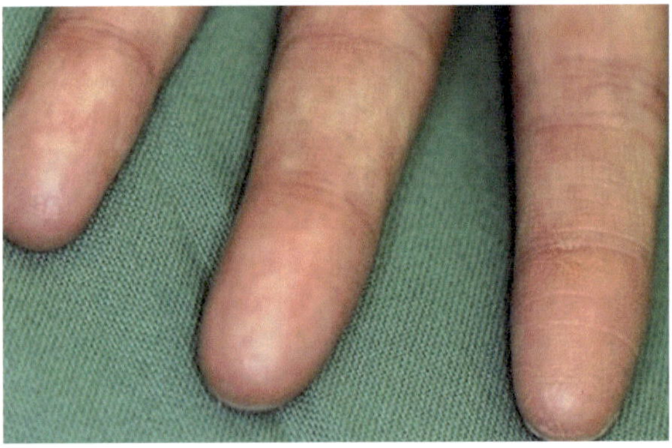

Fig. 3.3 Adermatoglyphia with an absence of loops, whorls, and arches that are present in normal fingertips (From Nousbeck et al. [6]. Copyright © 2011 The American Society of Human Genetics. Published by Elsevier Ltd. All right reserved)

Dermatoglyphs are an invaluable asset in identification of suspected individuals in the legal system. The microbiome, i.e. the group of living organisms, most notably the bacteria associated with the cutaneous tissue and these dermatoglyphs is not as well-known to the average juror, or used in the legal system. Each individual person is unique, as is their fingerprint, so what's not to say that their microbiome left behind on the fingerprint couldn't also be individualized? As opposed to other means of identification, which can be manipulated or may dissipate easily due to environmental conditions, bacteria tend to remain unaltered after an extended period of time. Also, in the field of forensic science, DNA of a suspect is difficult to recover unless there is a sufficient amount of bodily fluids or DNA-containing cells left at a crime scene. Bacteria are more resistant to temperature change, change in water or moisture content, and other variables, so a bacterial DNA that is associated with an individual could prove useful. Bacteria associated with the upper extremities and more specifically, the hands and fingers, are adept to living with the friction, chemical, and physical changes. Since bacteria frequently deal with these challenges, they are less likely to decrease in population over time. Since fingerprint damage easily occurs, whether intentional or accidental by the environment, or multiple people touching the same surface, a bacterial community left behind on an object may be more resistant to similar changes.

Using PCR of the 16sRNA gene sequences, a group of researchers Fierer et al. sequenced the bacterial communities found on computer mice and keyboards in a select group of individuals [10]. Statistical and algorithm analyses showed that the bacterial communities left on each keyboard and mouse greatly resembled the communities that were on the fingertips of each specific test subject. Across the bacterial communities of a previously established database, and across the other test participants in the study, the differences were significant. This research team was able to link each individual participant by their microbiome, or notably the bacterial communities, left behind on each keyboard and mouse to the microbiome of the cutaneous surface of participant's fingertips. This study was in a very isolated group however, and expansion across thousands of individuals and objects that are touched by multitudinous people may limit the ability of use on say, a door handle in an apartment building. However, using this analysis in the case of a robbery on a recovered. 45 caliber handgun where only few people have used the item could prove beneficial in selecting who had actually fired the weapon. This study also dictates than an object used by the same person frequently, like the keyboard or mouse, could be used in identification by their microbiome because the bacterial communities will be similar between the person's hands and the object.

Increased diversity in the microbiome of the upper extremities like the hands and fingers were further identified in a study by Fierer et al. [11] Bacterial swabs were performed on the hands of 51 individuals, 102 hands total. The 16sRNA genes were entered into a PCR sequence using a universal primer to mark the genes which enabled the ability to have one, single PCR sequence. Like the bacteria that normally reside on the epidermis, the phyla of organisms discovered most often to reside on the palmar surfaces of the test participants were *Proteobacteria*, *Actinobacteria*, and *Firmicutes* [11]. This study can aid in the future of forensic identification by the human microbiome due to the similarities and differences discovered in the palmar surfaces of all 102 hands. It was discovered the bacterial RNA present in the samples shared 5 bacterial phylotypes of the 4,742 total distinct phylotypes accounted for. This implies a vast amount of bacterial characteristic differences that exist between individuals listed in the group. There were also differences discovered in bacterial phylotypes between sex, hand-washing techniques and frequency, and intraindividual differences on the right hand vs the left hand depending on which hand was dominant, although the same hands on the same individual shared more commonalities than differences overall [11]. This study further verifies the potential for the bacterial communities of the epidermis and notably the upper extremities in forensic science.

However, in a criminal court case, a subject that is being investigated for a crime would have to be available for the microbiome to be used for identification. Since there is not a widely known database of every individual of the United States, or any country for that matter, for the current microbiome of each individual, limitations are bound to this technique. There is the Human Microbiome Project, which was funded to identify the microorganisms associated with health and disease in humans. The project was used to organize the bacterial cultures of 242 participants to represent the microbiome as a whole. The microbiome of individuals is not a readily tested methodology unlike fingerprints, which are used frequently in the criminal justice system. Limitations are exacerbated by a lack of database of these bacterial differences in individuals and this decreases the chances this system being used to identify a unique individual in a criminal case. Other limitations include frequency of exposure of an object to multiple people, and exactness of the technology to pinpoint a subject in a criminal court case as the legal system cannot rule on statistical probability of bacterial communities representing an individual like in the study by Fierer et al. [10].

The Human Microbiome and Assault

Every year there are over 293,000 sexual assault cases reported in the United States for victims over the age of 12, with every four out of five people knowing their attacker [12, 13]. According to the National Crime Victimization Survey during the years 2008–2012, 68 % of rape cases will go unreported to police, and roughly 98 % of cases will go without the attacker being incarcerated [14]. There are multiple variables as to why sexual assault cases have less chances of judicial success than other crimes. Forensic science relies on similar variables to armed robberies, homicide, assault and other crimes. These variables include body fluids like blood, saliva, semen, fecal matter, and other materials like dermatoglyphs, weapons, skin cells, hair, and visual identification. Using the bacterial communities of an attacker is a relatively new addition to the forensic scientist's tool belt.

In the case of any bodily intimate nature, whether it is kissing, sexual intercourse via genital, anal, or oral penetration; there is an exchange of fluids and those fluids will contain a bacterial populace that is unique to each individual involved. The bacterial populace can be present in but is not limited to: semen, saliva, blood, stool, vaginal secretions, epidermal cells of the genitals, and pubic hair follicles. Forensic scientists will also rely on similar bodily fluid exchange, even if by accident in any assault case.

Saliva

In different criminal court cases, like assault, sexual assault, and others, there is a likelihood of bodily fluid exchange. In cases of human bites, whether upon the attacker, or victim, there are bacterial communities that reside in the human mouth that carry their own DNA separate of the host. A bite does not need the amount of force to break the form of skin to cause injury or infection, but if the normal form of the skin is broken, bacterial infection chances increase dramatically. Bite marks used in the criminal justice system can be compared to the owner's teeth in a dental mold by a dentist or medical examiner. Limitations to using human saliva in a forensic laboratory on a victim comes down to timeliness, triage team and physician care after the incident, salivary enzymes that naturally can degrade the microbes, and integrity of the injury [15]. When a victim enters an emergency room or physician's office, it is up to the patient to notify the physicians that it was a human bite, and up to the physicians to take appropriate measures. The physicians should have access to a microbiology swab to take note of the saliva at the site of injury, and notify the police of the injury for forensic measures. According to a study by Patil et al., over 76 % of human bite injuries came to an emergency room under a 12-h window, with more than 77 % of all human bite patients receiving antibiotics as part of the medical treatment [15]. Since antibiotics have potential for exterminating foreign bacterial organisms coming from the suspect responsible for the bite, there should be a microbiology kit available. However a limitation to using bacteria transferred in a human bite comes down to the enzymes present in saliva that can degrade the bacteria before they can be cultured. Irrigating the site of injury and antibiotics are a core component to preventing bacterial infection of the bite, but in the case of a police investigation, microbiology samples should be a part of the triage process.

However, let's say we have access to the victim, the bite, and the bacteria left over from the saliva. Roughly 50 species of bacteria reside in the human saliva, with hundreds of millions of organisms overall [15]. *Staphylococcus*, *Streptococcus*, and *Eikenella* are the three bacteria known to be present in over half of all human bites, as they are part of the commensal species in human mouths. *Actinomyces*, *Neisseria*, and *Propionibacteria* are also considered to be core species that live in the human mouth. Research suggests that roughly 80 million bacteria are transferred in a 10-s kiss between two individuals, and that bacterial communities are similar between two partners that have oral embrace regularly than two strangers [16]. Using this data, a bacterial genome found in saliva at a crime scene or buccal swab could aid in possibly removing extraneous people, or including appropriate people from a suspect list. Certain bacteria that are common in disease and health states like *Candida albicans* are so common however, that identification by these species would be inadmissible in court.

Genitalia, Anal Tissue, Stool

The genital and anal regions of the body contain a very separate microbiome of viruses and bacteria than the torso, extremities, and face (Fig. 3.4). The genital and anal areas are susceptible to unique bacteria, fungi, and viruses transmitted by sexual contact and fluid exchange. The human male and female both share hair strands located in the perianal and genital regions of the body, with bacterial changes associated with their

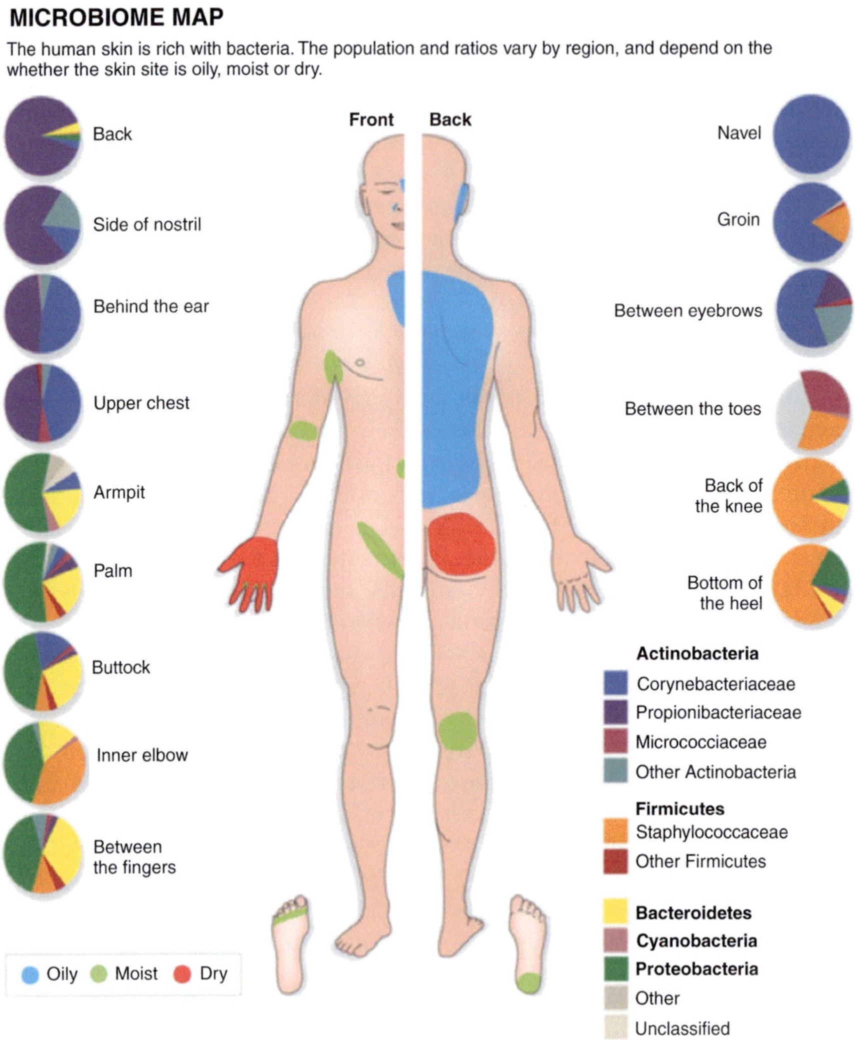

Fig. 3.4 A map of the microbiome of the skin listed by region of the human body (With permission from Trivedi [26]. © Nature Publishing Group)

daily local environments. For instance, since women are more likely to partake in grooming techniques in the genital regions, the commensal bacteria present will be species that can survive in a grooming environment. However, in only about 4 % of sexual assault cases are pubic hair strands recovered at a crime scene or on the victim in a crime [17]. They also are relatively difficult to garner nuclear DNA from due to the forensic science reliance on Short Tandem Repeat analysis. However, a study revealed that using Next Generation Sequencing and Metagenomics can aid in using the bacterial genomefound on pubic hairs and hairs on the scalp [17].

Present research and medical professionals agree that one of the dominant bacteria present in the genitals for the human female is *Lactobacillus*, which could be a suitable marker that bacteria left behind containing higher amounts of *Lactbacillus* would be female. The same research by Tridico et al. show that men contain higher amounts of transient bacteria in the groin region than women do [17]. The opposite was found in scalp bacteria as where women had higher amounts of transient bacteria than men do, which is possibly secondary to higher percentiles of different grooming techniques in women. Also, women had more distinct communities of bacteria in the groin and scalp region than men did overall. Permanent residents on the scalp were identified as *Anaerococcus* and transient members included of *Knoellia* species.

In a case of sexual assault between, let's say male and female, there is potential for exchange of the bacteria that reside in both male and female, and even more likelihood of exchange if no sexual barrier like a condom is used. Research from Tridico et al. suggest that persistence of the suspect's bacterial identity and its persistence in the victim's genitals would be the most useful marker in identification, were the bacterial genome to be used in a criminal court case. Timeliness of triage by hospital staff, microbiology, and police are important in taking samples of the bacteria present. Other important aspects to consider are the suspect's bacterial reports if the suspect is known, and genital microbiology of the current sexual partner of the victim. While nuclear DNA is difficult to garner from pubic and scalp hairs, the bacteria present and their DNA is not. While bacteria on the scalp might be more temporally diverse due to multitudinous microbial exposure, the genitals tend to be isolated to their local environment and thus, more susceptible to maintaining a relatively unwavering bacterial community. In the research by Tridico et al. there were differences in noted between scalp hair and genital hair follicles in regards to bacterial communities. While scalp hair contained roughly 50 bacterial species for men, and 55 for women, genital hair follicles contained roughly 73 species for men and 76 for women. This implies potential for differentiation between pubic hair and scalp hair, and sexual identities based on numbers of species alone. It was also revealed in the study performed there were similarities in two participant's pubic bacterial communities that were cohabitating, and also had sexual relations before the study was performed [17].

Sexually transmitted bacteria and infections rely on sexual contact and fluid exchange whether it is genital, anal, or oral. Three common bacteria involved in sexually transmitted diseases are *Neisseria gonorrhoeae*, *Chlamydia gonorrhoeae*, and *Treponema pallidum*, the bacteria that cause gonorrhea, chlamydia, and syphillus respectively. These bacteria contain their own nuclear DNA but can be difficult to track due to the sheer amount of people that contract these bacteria and their infections each year. This would become a piece circumstantial evidence, and proving the disease to be contacted through sexual misconduct would be difficult. In a situation where a person under the legal age of sexual consent has contracted one of these infections, a bacterial comparison by genotype could be conducted as someone regardless of circumstances cannot consent to any form of sexual activity [18]. A similar case was tried and convicted a criminal accused of sexual misconduct with a minor (someone under the age of sexual consent) using similar circumstances with *N. gonorrhea*. The suspect was convicted by a comparison of his strain of *N. gonorrhea* found on his clothing and the victim's strain [19].

Recently an advanced strain of *N. gonorrhea* was identified in Japan in 2011 and it was found to be antibiotic resistant [20]. Resistance stems from different factors like increased dependence on penicillin, transmission of the bacteria in people who go untreated for lengthy periods of time, efflux pumps in the bacteria that aid in defense against modern medications, chromosomal changes in the genome of the bacteria, and people who are treated multiple times for the disease after transmission [21]. A super-strain of *N. gonorrhea* is a rare strain of bacteria that is resistant to the tetracyclins and β-lactamase inhibitors used in primary bacterial infections. In a case where a victim develops antibiotic-resistant gonorrhea and a suspect is discovered, a comparison of the strain of *N. gonorrhoeae* in the victim and suspect could aid in a criminal court decision.

Human stool is generally a well-preserved interpretation of the bacterial and viral species that reside in the gastrointestinal tract. Using PCR methods, these microbes that are responsible for the health and pathology associated with the GI tract can be isolated and solidified. Organisms present in the stool have varying places of origin, like the epithelium or endothelium, and can be indicators of diseases like gastroenteritis or colon cancer (Fig. 3.5) [22].

A research study performed by Franzosa et al., using the Human Microbiome Project information and a mathematic algorithm to identify 242 individuals by their

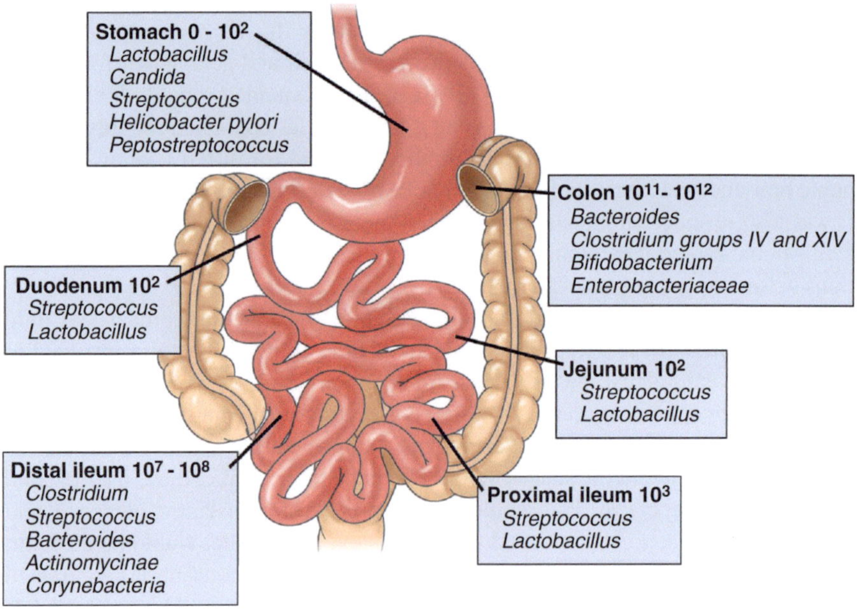

Fig. 3.5 Composition and luminal concentrations of dominant microbial species in various regions of the gastrointestinal tract (With permission from Sartor [27]. © Elsevier)

microbiomes in the Human Microbiome Project. The highest match rate with correct identification was by the microbiomes present in stool samples by 86 %, with the least number of identified individuals in skin cells [23]. While stool does carry a significant amount of human nuclear DNA due to white blood cells, another proportion of DNA in stool would be due to bacteria. Stool is already used today as a method of DNA authentication in forensic science, but the study by Franzosa et al. shows promise in suspect identification in the legal system using different microbial organisms' DNA. Due to chemical and environmental factors, human DNA may be difficult to extract from stool samples. Bacteria, however, tend to remain longer in dried samples of stool and might be more resistant to environmental challenges. In a case of assault or neglect; bacterial cultures have shown to have promise in accurate human identification via stool samples.

Conclusion

Since the advent of the Human Microbiome Project, where the bacterial DNA and bacterial identities were found and organized into an entire database, the use of the human microbiome has been extensive in clinical, educational, and legal settings. Research studies have used the database to identify significant bacterial changes in the vaginal tissue during pregnancy, and have also used it to identify humans by comparisons of their present bacterial communities, to those listed on the database [24]. This opens a new door of identification and prosecution for members in the legal and forensic services. While nuclear human DNA is an invaluable source, it may not always be available, due to temporal or environmental limitations. Bacterial DNA and bacterial cultures tend to be more resistant to environmental and temporal challenges experienced in the field or as a part of human tissue, and this is creates the interest in research for forensic science. Using bacterial differences between people may be hindered by current limitations in the legal system, however. Statistical analyses, reliance on the suspect's presence in an investigation, and similarities between individuals' microbiome are challenges that await in the legal and forensic system. However, with techniques noted in Fierer et al., there is promise for using the organisms that reside on and around people everyday [11].

References

1. Forensic. (n.d.). In Oxford dictionaries online. Retrieved from http://www.oxforddictionaries.com/us/definition/american_english/forensic.
2. Ruitberg CM, Reeder DJ, Butler JM. STRBase: a short tandem repeat DNA database for the human identity testing community. Nucleic Acids Res. 2001;29(1):320–2.
3. National Forensic Science Technology Center® (n.d.) Crime scene investigator- a simplified guide to fingerprint analysis. Retrieved from http://www.crime-scene-investigator.net/SimplifiedGuideFingerprints.pdf.

4. Shepherd R. Simpson's forensic medicine (2003). New York: Oxford University Press; 2003. p. 34–50, 60–8, 94–102, 10–3.
5. Reddy K, Lowenstein E. Forensics in dermatology: part I. J Am Acad Dermatol. 2011;64(5):801–8.
6. Nousbeck J, Burger B, Fuchs-Telem D, Pavlovsky M, Fenig S, Sarig O, et al. A mutation in a skin-specific isoform of SMARCAD1 causes autosomal-dominant adermatoglyphia. Am J Hum Genet. 2011;89(2):302–7. doi:10.1016/j.ajhg.2011.07.004.
7. Heimer W, Brauner G, James W. Dermatopathia pigmentosa reticularis: a report of a family demonstrating autosomal dominant inheritance. J Am Acad Dermatol. 1992;26(2):298–301.
8. Komatz Y, Yoshida O. Finger patterns and ridge counts of patients with Klinefelter's syndrome (47, XXY) among the Japanese. Hum Hered. 1976;26:290–7.
9. Rajangam S, Janakiram S, Thomas I. Dermatoglyphics in Down's syndrome. J Indian Med Assoc. 1995;93(1):10–3.
10. Fierer N, Lauber C, Zhou N, McDonald D, Costello E, Knight R. From the cover: forensic identification using skin bacterial communities. Proc Natl Acad Sci. 2010;107(14):6477–81.
11. Fierer N, Hamady M, Lauber C, Knight R. The influence of Sex, handedness, and washing on the diversity of hand surface bacteria. Proc Natl Acad Sci. 2008;105(46):17994–9.
12. Hannigan G, Grice E. Microbial ecology of the skin in the era of metagenomics and molecular microbiology. Cold Spring Harbor Perspect Med. 2013;3(12):1–4.
13. How often does sexual assault occur? | RAINN | Rape, Abuse and Incest National Network, 2013. Retrieved August 4, 2015.
14. Truman J, Planty M. Criminal victimization, 2011. NCJ Bulletin 2012. Retrieved from August 4, 2015. http://www.bjs.gov/content/pub/pdf/cv11.pdf.
15. Patil P, Panchabhai T, Galwankar S. Managing human bites. J Emerg Trauma Shock. 2009;2(3):186.
16. Kort R, Caspers M, Graaf A, Egmond W, Keijser B, Roeselers G. Shaping the oral microbiota through intimate kissing. Microbiome. 2014;2:1–41.
17. Tridico S, Murray D, Addison J, Kirkbride K, Bunce M. Metagenomic analyses of bacteria on human hairs: a qualitative assessment for applications in forensic science. Invest Genet. 2014;5:1–16.
18. Gunn A, Sarah P. Microbes as forensic indicators. Trop Biomed. 2012;29(3):311–30.
19. Martin I, Foreman E, Hall V, Nesbitt A, Forster G, Ison C. Non-cultural detection and molecular genotyping of Neisseria gonorrhoeae from a piece of clothing. J Med Microbiol. 2007;56:487–90.
20. Ohnishi M, Saika T, Hoshina S, Iwasaku K, Nakayama S, Watanabe H, et al. Ceftriaxone-resistant Neisseria gonorrhoeae, Japan. Emerg Infect Dis. 2011;17(1):148–9.
21. Levy S, Marshall B. Antibacterial resistance worldwide: causes, challenges and responses. Nat Med. 2004;10(12):S122–9.
22. Sonke E, Haj-Ahmad Y. Detection of viral, bacterial and human genomic DNA from preserved stool samples. 2013. Retrieved August 7, 2015. https://norgenbiotek.com/sites/default/files/resources/stool_dna_isolation_kit_detection_of_viral_bacterial_and_human_genomic_dna_from_preserved_stool_samples_application_notes_51.pdf.
23. Franzosa E, Huang K, Meadow J, Gevers D, Lemon K, Bohannan B, et al. Identifying personal microbiomes using metagenomic codes. Proc Natl Acad Sci U S A. 2005;112(22):1–2.
24. Aagaard K, Riehle K, Ma J, Segata N, Mistretta T-A, Coarfa C, et al. A metagenomic approach to characterization of the vaginal microbiome signature in pregnancy. PLoS One. 2012;7(6):e36466.
25. Coren S. Searching for genetic markers for specific behaviors: a group technique to assess fingerprint patterns. Bull Psychonomic Soc. 1987;25(2):82–4.
26. Trivedi B. Microbiome: the surface brigade. Nature. 2012;491:S60–1.
27. Sartor R. Microbial influences in inflammatory Bowel diseases. Gastroenterology. 2008;134(2):577–94.

Chapter 4
Dermatopathology, Genetics, and Intergenerational Dermatology

Robert A. Norman and Lauren M. Murray

Abstract Dermatopathology is a field of dermatology that is becoming increasingly important. It allows practitioners to have more precision with their diagnoses through the use of various staining. Advancements in genetics have also allowed for possible new therapy and treatments of different dermatologic cancers and diseases based on targeting specific gene mutations. In being able to better understand the location and types of changes in a person's genome, physicians will be able to more readily differentiate between different subtypes of specific pathologies and provide more personalized treatment options.

Keywords Dermatopathology • Genetics • Skin • Cancer • Genodermatoses • Future • Intergenerational Dermatology

Dermatopathology

Dermatopathology uses histology to help dermatopathologists come to a precise diagnosis of a dermatologic sample [1]. They use the microscope, both electron and light, to evaluate these samples along with the use of immunohistochemistry and histochemical stains, immunofluorescence, and many other techniques to evaluate the samples provided to the lab. Many of these stains can help the dermatopathologist or pathologist identify antigens, organisms, and cell types within the samples [2]. This can help with further evaluation of the sample and help lead to a better more specific diagnosis, whether it be a malignancy, congenital skin pathology, or acquired skin pathology. According to the American Academy of Dermatology,

R.A. Norman, DO, MPH, MBA (✉)
Dermatology Healthcare, 8002 Gunn Highway, Tampa, FL 33626, USA

Professor, Department of Dermatology, Nova Southeastern Medical School, Ft. Lauderdale, FL, USA
e-mail: skindrrob@aol.com

L.M. Murray, OMS, IV
Department of Dermatology, Nova Southeastern University, Tampa, FL, USA

R.A. Norman (ed.), *Personalized, Evolutionary, and Ecological Dermatology*,
DOI 10.1007/978-3-319-41088-3_4

dermatopathologists have extensive training in evaluation of skin tissue samples from dermatology patients [3].

Currently, the biopsy is the test of choice for diagnosis and confirmation of numerous dermatological processes. Although the biopsy is a very affective means for diagnosing pathology, it is an invasive procedure, which can lead to scarring of the patient's skin. Crowsen, in one of his articles, discusses the possibility of non-invasive techniques in dermatology for the diagnosis of different skin pathologies that may be available in the future [4]. One of these techniques includes near-infrared spectroscopy. Near-infrared spectroscopy allows the physician to look at the specimen in real time without having to cut into the patient's skin via a fiberoptic device that measures reflected light. In Crowsen's study, the near-infrared spectroscopy was able to correctly identify dysplastic nevi from banal nevi 97.7 % of the time. However, in regards to being able to identify a dysplastic nevi from a seborrheic keratosis the near-infrared spectroscopy had only a 72.4 % accuracy [4]. Hopefully, further advancements in technology and more studies performed in the use of near-infrared spectroscopy as a non-invasive procedure for identifying skin pathology will allow for this technique to be used in dermatology clinics.

With the increased number of patients living into the geriatric age range, the number of patients with dermatologic complaints will continue to increase [5]. This ever-growing patient population, coupled with the increasing number of biopsies performed yearly by dermatologists, will fuel the need for board certified dermatopathologists. Currently, in some countries such as Japan, there is a shortage of physicians trained in dermatopathology to help interpret the histological findings of dermatology patients' biopsies [5]. Dermatologists must continue to find more inventive ways to have their biopsies read in a timely, cost-effective manner.

One study focused on a potential use of online consultation service using virtual slides to help with this shortage in physicians specialized in dermatopathology [5]. One of the limitations of using telepathology was the lack of ability to magnify or focus the virtual slide [5]. The study mentioned the classic whole slide image has better magnification and focus; however, hopefully, with the advances in technology and better availability of telepathology it may become a more cost effective option in terms of looking at histological specimens. The study suggested the use of telepathology might help eliminate shipping costs and be more convenient for the dermatopathologist who is reading the sample [5].

Studies have also looked at the use of smartphone applications to help dermatopathologists with visualizations of different skin pathologies [6]. One study discussed how the use of medical applications of smartphones in different fields of medicine has been increasing; however, there is currently no monitoring body over these applications so users must be aware of the products they are using [6]. The study alluded to how fields of medicine that rely on visualization could find these applications very useful in the future.

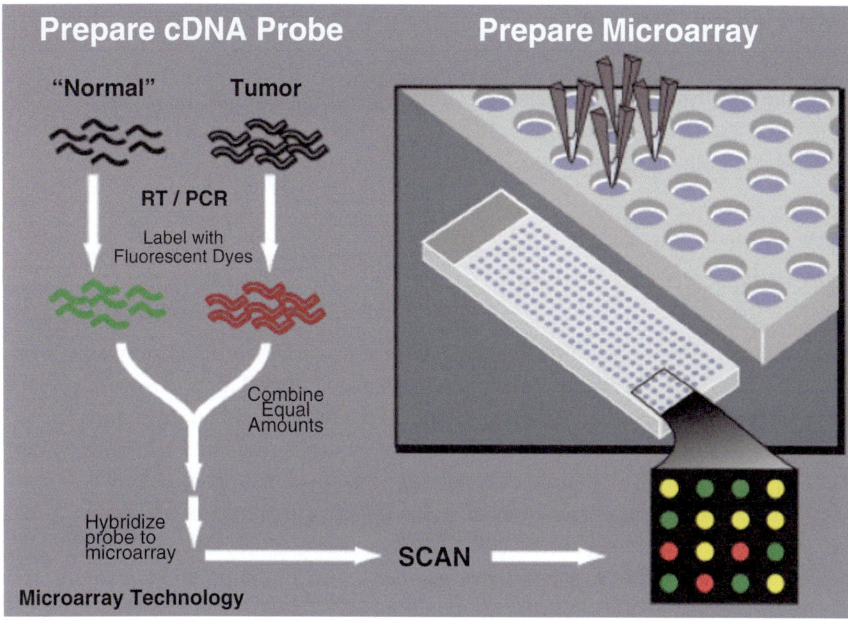

Fig. 4.1 Complementary DNA microarray – National Human Genome Research Institute. *Microarray Technology*; 2015 (Available at: https://www.genome.gov/10000533. Accessed October 9, 2015. Courtesy: National Human Genome Research Institute)

Genetics

Genetics have begun to play a larger role in medicine as the human genome becomes better understood. As there are greater advancements in the fields of genetics, there will be better understanding between pathology and the genes associated with specific cancers and diseases.

According to Crowen, the Human Genome Project had identified over 25,000 unique genes [4]. Complementary DNA microarray has become a way for scientists to visualize the levels of gene transcription in a sample. This information can then be used to compare the gene transcription levels of normal skin versus that in different pathological processes. One study discussed unpublished data on the use of microarray to look at the upregulation of eight different genes in basal cell carcinoma compared to normal skin (Fig. 4.1) [4].

There is currently advanced research being done in regards to gene therapy for treatment of different skin diseases, aiming to treat some of the changes that occur secondary to gene mutations [7]. Hopefully sometime in the near future these treatments will improve and different skin diseases will be able to be treated with a customized therapy based on the patient's specific genetic mutation or changes.

Skin Cancer

According to the Center for Disease Control, skin cancers are the most common form of cancer in the United States [8]. Non-epithelial skin cancers, including basal cell and squamous cell carcinoma of the skin, account for 7 % of all cancers [8].

Squamous Cell Carcinoma

Squamous cell carcinoma of the skin is classified as a non-epithelial skin cancer [8]. It is the second most common tumor of sun-exposed areas [7]. It is uncommon for these tumors to metastasize. Histologically, theses tumors, including squamous cell carcinoma in situ, have enlarged, hyperchromic nuclei throughout the entire epidermis [7]. There can also be large areas of keratinization, with some being so undifferentiated that immunohistochemical stains for keratin are needed to confirm that the cancer is actually a squamous cell [7].

There appears to be an association between a *p53* mutation and squamous cell carcinoma. Multiple other cancers are thought to be associated with a p53 mutation [7, 9]. When the *p53* gene is not functioning correctly, the DNA damaged induced by UV light may not be properly repaired. The process leads to cells with errors in their DNA sequence, which are passed on to their daughter cells and can eventually lead to a cancerous process [7]. A study by Brash found 58 % of invasive squamous cell carcinomas of the skin had mutations of the *p53* gene [9]. These mutations altered the amino acid sequence in the genome [9].

Basal Cell Carcinoma

Basal cell carcinoma is the most common malignancy amongst white skinned individuals [10, 11]. Similar to squamous cell carcinoma of the skin, basal cell carcinoma rarely metasizes [7]. Patients with basal cell carcinoma are at increased risk of developing basal cell carcinoma again or other types of skin cancers [12].

Histologically, these tumor cells look similar to the basal cells of the epidermis [7]. They can grow in a multifocal way, starting in the dermis and growing outwards, or in a nodular pattern, growing into the dermis. According to Maloney, basal cell carcinomas have a "classic" histopathology [11]. In one of her articles, she describes the histopathology of basal cell carcinoma as having "individual basaloid cells that are uniform and have a bland or nonanaplastic appearance, peripheral palisading of basophilic tumor islands, and retraction of the surround stroma from the tumor islands." [11] There are also several histological subtypes of basal cell carcinoma including nodular and superficial [11].

There have been several genes found to be associated with basal cell carcinoma. Nevoid basal cell carcinoma syndrome is inherited in an autosomal dominant pattern [7]. Patients are born with a mutation in the *PTCH* gene on chromosome 9q22.3 [7, 12]. Usually a second form of injury, sometimes in the form of UV light, is needed to knock out the second normal allele, which leads to the development of this syndrome [7].

PTCH mutations have been found in 20 % of sporadic basal cell carcinomas [7]. Another gene mutation implicated in the development of basal cell carcinoma is the *p53* gene mutation. Mutation in the *p53* gene can be seen in 40–60 % of basal cell carcinoma [7]. As discussed above, *p53* mutations can be caused by exposure to UV light.

Melanoma

According to the American Academy of Dermatology the incidence of melanoma in the United States has doubled between 1982 and 2011 [13]. Caucasian males over 50 appear to be at the highest risk for the development of melanoma [13]. Recognition of melanoma early is extremely important because unlike squamous cell carcinoma of the skin and basal cell carcinoma, melanomas tend to metastasize early. They are usually resistant to treatment as well [7]. Melanoma makes up approximately 1.7 % of all cancer related deaths [14].

Melanomas typically have a radial and vertical growth phase. Histologically, the radial growth phase has nests of cells with melanocytes in the epidermis [7]. During the vertical phase, which is the more dangerous and concerning phase, nodularity of the infiltrating cells becomes apparent on histology [7].

Outcome measures for melanoma can be predicted based off histology [7]. For example, the probability of metastasis can be correlated to the depth at which the melanoma has invaded [7]. Also, the number of mitoses seen on histology has been correlated with the outcome of the disease [7].

Genetics also play an important factor in the development of melanomas. Several genes have been implemented in the development of melanoma. Some of these genes include: *MC1R, ASIP, TYR, RB* tumor suppressors gene, *CDK 4/6, CDKN2A* [7, 15]. The CDKN2A gene is mutated in approximately 40 % of patients with autosomal dominant familial melanoma and about 10 % of sporadic melanoma [7]. It is also the strongest risk factor in the development of melanoma [15]. *RB* mutations are also seen in both familial and sporadic melanomas [7].

With advancements in gene analysis, it is hoped that someday in the future patients will be able to know their risk of developing melanoma [15]. Since there are numerous different genetic mutations that have been found to be associated with the development of melanoma, there have been attempts at developing therapies that target some of the changes on the molecular level the genes mutations cause [7]. Hopefully in the future, these treatments will be deemed successful and can be implemented into use for treatment of melanoma.

Genodermatoses

Geneodermatoses are genetic conditions that are associated with genetic syndromes [16]. Many of these diseases follow Mendelian genetics and are inherited in an autosomal dominant or recessive or X-linked dominant or recessive pattern [7, 16]. There are numerous geneodermatoses and they can be diagnosed based on clinical features, labs, histology, and molecular analysis [16]. It is important to identify these patients with geneodermatoses because of the genetic components of the diseases. The numerous geneodermatoses are subdivided into multiple categories; however, this chapter will focus on several of the more common geneodermatoses.

Neurofibromatosis

There are two different types of neurofibromatosis, type 1 (NF1) and type 2 (NF2). They are both inherited in an autosomal dominant pattern [7]. NF1 is more common than NF2.

NF1 is caused by issues with the NF1 gene, which is located at chromosome 17q11.2. This gene is very large and codes for neurofbromin [7]. It is difficult to pinpoint an exact mutation in the NF1 gene given there have been 2030 genetic mutations recorded for the NF1 gene based on information provided by the Human Gene Mutation Database [17]. Clinically, NF1 presents with neurofibromas, which can appear on the skin, optic nerve gliomas, Lisch nodules, and café au lait spots. Diagnosis of NF1 is typically made using the National Health Institute criteria for NF1.

NF2 is also inherited in an autosomal dominant patter but is much less common than NF1. The NF2 gene is located on chromosome 22q12, which codes for the merlin, a tumor suppressor gene [7]. Clinically, NF2 presents with cranial nerve 8 schwannomas, usually bilateral, meningiomas, gliomas, as well as café au lait spots (Figs. 4.2 and 4.3) [7].

Tuberous Sclerosis

Tuberous sclerosis is another disease that is inherited in an autosomal dominant pattern. These patients typically have harmatomas and other neoplasms of the brain, heart, eye, kidney and skin [18]. The cutaneous findings associated with this disease include angiofibromas (Fig. 4.4), shargreen patches (Fig. 4.5), ash-leaf patches (Fig. 4.6), and subungal fibromas [7].

There two major genes associated with tuberous sclerosis. These genes include TSC1, found on chromosome 9q34, which encodes for hamartin, and TSC2, which is located on chromosome 16p13.3 and encodes for tuberin [7]. Of these two mutations the TSC2 mutation is more common [7]. Tuberin and hamartin work as a herterodimer to help suppress mTOR signaling [18].

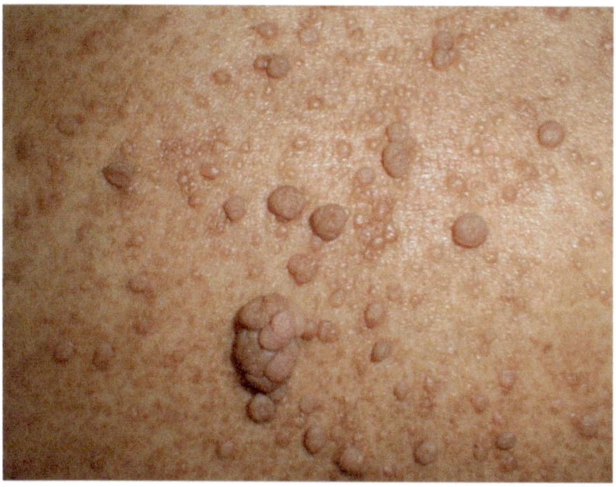

Fig. 4.2 Neurofibromas – UCSD. *Neurofibromas.*; 2005 (Available at: https://meded.ucsd.edu/clinicalimg/skin_neurofibroma.htm. Accessed October 12, 2015. Copyright ©2015, The Regents of the University of California. All rights reserved. Last updated 10/15)

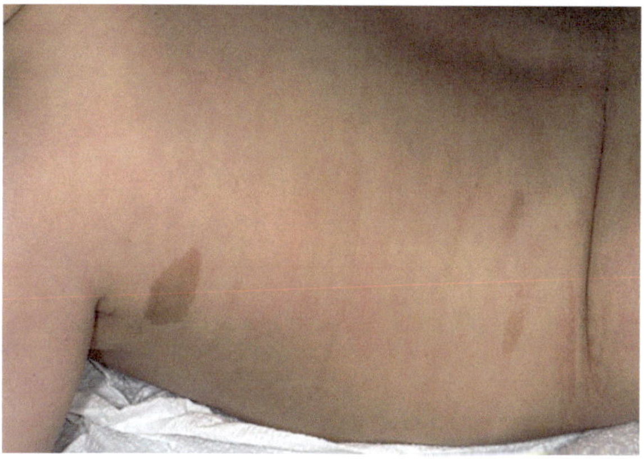

Fig. 4.3 Café au lait spots – Webmd. *Cafe-Au-Lait Spots.*; 2007 (Available at: http://www.webmd.com/skin-problems-and-treatments/picture-of-cafe-au-lait-spots. Accessed October 12, 2015. ©2013, WebMD, LLC. All rights reserved)

Xeroderma Pigmentosum

Xeroderma pigmentosum (XP) is a rare autosomal recessive disease. This disorder is caused by mutations in the genes that are involved in DNA repair. XP was the first DNA-repair disorder to be discovered [19]. Because of this mutation, people with XP are extremely sensitive to UV light. The cutaneous manifestations can range from cancer to freckles [19]. There are eight different subgroupings of XP titled XP-A through XP-G along with XP-variant [19]. There are also eight genes that

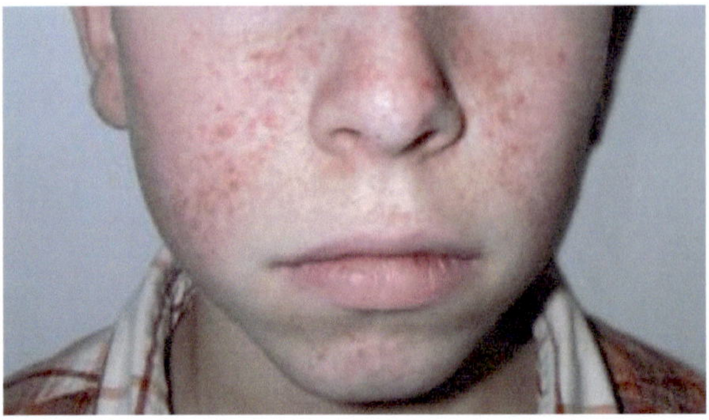

Fig. 4.4 Angiofibromas – CHOP. *Angiofibromas.*; 2013 (Available at: http://www.chop.edu/conditions-diseases/angiofibromas#.Vhr58BNViko. Accessed October 12, 2015. © 1996–2014 by The Children's Hospital of Philadelphia. All rights reserved)

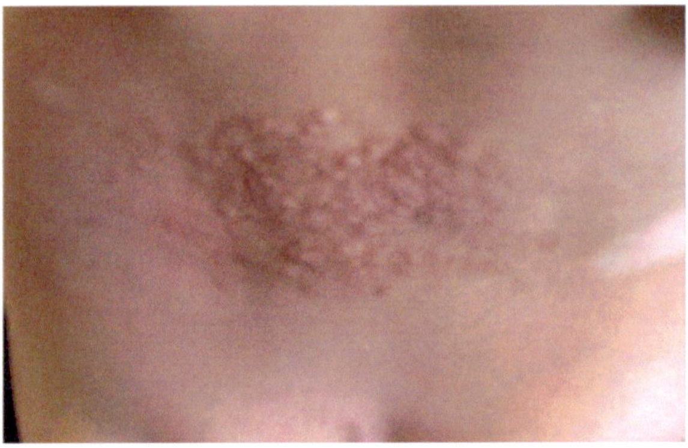

Fig. 4.5 Shagreen Patch-Mass General. *Shagreen Patches.*; 2006 (Available at: http://www2.massgeneral.org/livingwithtsc/affects/skin.htm. Accessed October 12, 2015. © 2006 The General Hospital Corporation)

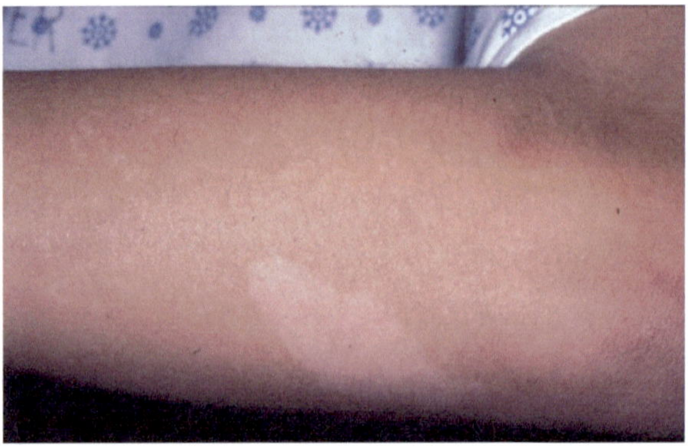

Fig. 4.6 Ash-Leaf spot – UCSF. *Ash Leaf Macule* (Available at: http://missinglink.ucsf.edu/lm/DermatologyGlossary/ash_leaf_macule.html. Accessed October 12, 2015. © The Regents of the University of California, 2015)

have been discovered to cause XP. They are DDB2, ERCC2, ERCC3, ERCC4, ERCC5, POLH, XPA, and XPC (Fig. 4.7) [20].

Basal Cell Nevus Syndrome

Basal cell nevus syndrome (BCNS) is an autosomal dominant disorder that causes multiple basal cell carcinomas (Fig. 4.8) [7]. It is also known as Gorlin syndrome [7]. The disorder is associated with a mutation in PTCH, which is located on chromosome 9q22.3 [7]. People with BCNS are born with one defective copy of the PTCH1 gene [21, 22]. Since this is a heredity disorder, it is encouraged the affected person see a geneticist [22].

Clinically, the patients can have other tumors, intracranial calcification, cleft lip/palate, and rib abnormalities [7]. The basal cell carcinomas usually begin to appear between puberty and age 35 with the most common locations being the face, back, and neck [22].

Intergenerational Dermatology

Here I (RAN) introduce the concept of Intergenerational Dermatology. The field of Intergenerational Dermatology lives in the interweaving of biological, cultural, economic, psychological and epigenetic components of our lives. I have emphasized

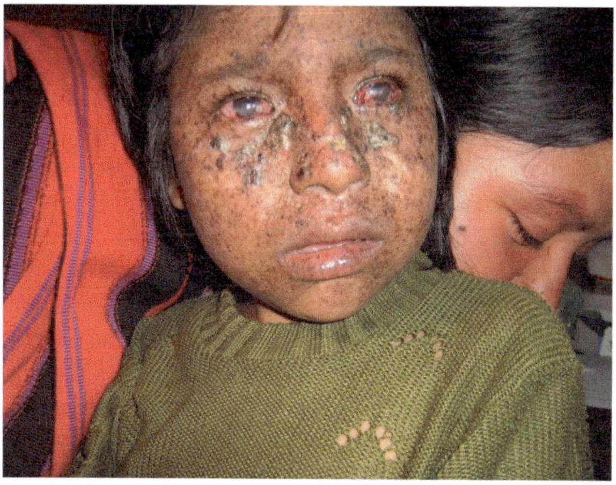

Fig. 4.7 Xeroderma pigmentosum (From Halpern et al. [21] Copyright © 2008 Halpern et al.; licensee BioMed Central Ltd. This is an Open Access article distributed under the terms of the Creative Commons Attribution License (http://creativecommons.org/licenses/by/2.0), which permits unrestricted use, distribution, and reproduction in any medium, provided the original work is properly cited)

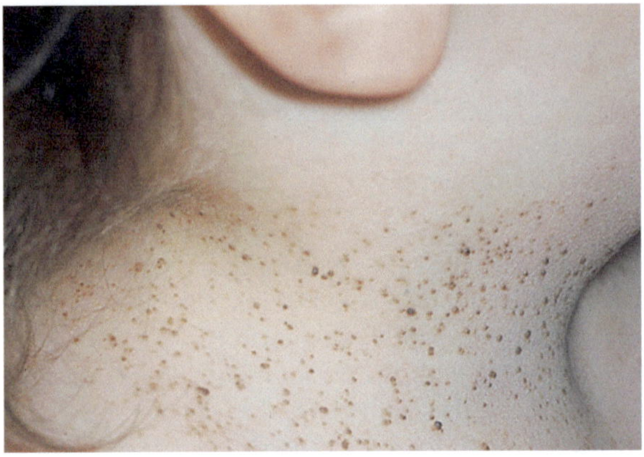

Fig. 4.8 Basal Cell Nevus Syndrome. 13. Webmd. *Basal Cell Nevus Syndrome*.; 2014 (Available at: http://www.webmd.com/skin-problems-and-treatments/picture-of-basal-cell-nevus-syndrome. Accessed October 12, 2015. © 2005–2015 WebMD, LLC. All rights reserved)

generational topics in detail in my books on geriatrics, preventive and integrative dermatology, and continue to emphasize how small changes in behavior and exposures can affect one's whole life and subsequent generations. I am now expanding this concept to a much bigger and more ambitious picture, from the beginning of our existence as humans and telescoping into the future.

Intergenerational Medicine is in its infancy, with the field of epigenetics being used as a springboard for further research. The concept includes the newest data and research in general dermatology, pediatric dermatology, geriatric dermatology and all branches of medicine.

Infectious diseases, especially in pregnant women, may affect subsequent generations in reproductive capacity, long-term morbidity and economic disruption. Conflicts that result in interruptions in education (a chronic atopic or Epidermolysis bullosa child missing weeks of school) may lessen skills and knowledge in vulnerable children and consequently deplete resources from society.

Over time a person may be influenced by good or bad habits and actions at a young age, often influenced by his or her family of origin. An example would be applying sun blocks when young and having an absence of skin cancers later in life. The effects of biology, culture, psychology, demographics, and economics on skin and general health for us and our offspring include ways an individual can make positive changes for subsequent generations based on actions that elicit protein changes effecting RNA and DNA. Patient compliance with medicine usage and healthy behavior make an imprint deep in the genetic level.

In similar fashion, smoking or poor nutritional habits based on poor life choices, economic inadequacies, and genetic mismatches may manifest in both personal and intergenerational mishap. When you counsel a patient on eradicating detrimental habits and emphasizing beneficial ones, you are counseling an entire genetic line of *Homo sapiens*.

Certain articles have sprung up on Intergenerational Medicine. Included are Devakumar et al's article examining the intergenerational effects of four features of conflict: violence, challenges to mental health, infection and malnutrition [23]. The authors document the short- and medium-term effects of conflict on population health and its consequences across generations and potential harms to the health of children yet to be born. Wong et al. described intergenerational transmission of pathogenic heteroplasmic mitochondrial DNA in a study on the pattern of intergenerational transmission of pathogenic mitochondrial DNA [24]. Whitaker et al. has published on the intergenerational transmission of thinness [25].

Intergenerational Dermatology is an exciting and provocative subject within dermatology and I believe should be embraced by all practitioners who want to fully care for each patient and see the big picture that occurs with each patient interaction.

The Future

In *The Future Direction of Dermatologic Therapy* and *The Blue Man* I and certain contributors proposed some insight into the potential technology that could be used in the field of dermatology in the future [26, 27]. As far as detection, there will be computers and robots that will do full-body scans on a semi-annual basis and be able to compare changes in moles or other concerning external and internal developments. Physicians will be there to verify these findings, biopsy as necessary, and initiate treatment.

New devices to detect skin cancer and other skin maladies include Image Analysis and Computer –assisted Diagnosis, Multispectral Imaging and Automated Diagnosis, Confocal laser microscopy, optical coherence tomography, ultrasound, MRI, spectrophotometric intracutaneous analysis, and artificial neural networks. Continuous research and refinement will allow improvements in detection and treatment.

Armed with hand-held spectrophotometric and chemical detection devices the vast majority of cutaneous neoplasms will not only be accurately identified but risk assessed in situ. Characteristic light diffraction spectra will differentially fingerprint the types of cutaneous malignancy and the application of light or sound emitting devices will precisely gauge the depth of tumor penetration. Chemical detecting devices programmed to recognize subtle changes in the metabolic by-products of cancerous cells will complement the light-emitting devices. Similarly, these devices will be relied upon to assess the extent of residual disease. Computerized algorithms that reconcile the measured variables of epidermal thickness, vascular density and depth of inflammatory infiltrate with pre-programmed archetypes will also permit the assessment and identification of many dermatoses. Such advances will undoubtedly change the role of and importance of dermatopathology in the equation of dermatologic care as they may be relegated to the arbitration of equivocal cases or sought in the assessment of confounding data or following incomplete response to therapy. For questionable diagnoses, teledermatopathology referral to other specialists will be utilized.

Conclusion

Dermatopathology and genetics are two very important parts of the field of dermatology. Both allow physicians to be better able to diagnose and treat their patients more appropriately. Dermatopathology gives a better look at what is happening in the skin at a microscopic level. It allows the dermatopathologist or pathologist to better identify the cause of the patient's lesion. With further advances in staining along with other forms of technology such virtual slides, non-invasive techniques, and smartphone applications it will be interesting to see what the future holds in regards to the number of punch and shave biopsies and frozen sections performed in the dermatology office and what new advancements in the skin field will be made over the next few decades. Other questions to consider with these advances in technology is how will cost affect these procedures and how will they be reimbursed via insurance companies.

The genetic aspect of dermatology is particularly up and coming. With further advances in genetic profiling, physicians will be better suited to treat many of the dermatologic pathologies. In regards to these ailments, research is being conducted to target these genetic changes in hopes that treatments geared toward mutations can help stop the process. When this happens, patients will essentially be able to have treatments customized towards their skin ailment that reflect their own genome.

References

1. Bergman R. Dermatopathology and molecular genetics. J Am Acad Dermatol. 2008;58(3):452–7. doi:10.1016/j.jaad.2007.12.008.
2. Soeprono F. A systematic approach to dermatopathology. Loma Linda: Loma Linda University Printing Services; 2006.
3. Aad.org. What is a dermatopathologist? 2015. Available at: https://www.aad.org/dermatology-a-to-z/about-dermatology/what-is-a-dermatopathologist. Accessed 6 Oct 2015.
4. Crowson A. The future of dermatopathology. Mod Pathol. 2005. doi:10.1038/modpathol.3800513.
5. Nakayama I, Matsumura T, Kamataki A, et al. Development of a teledermatopathology consultation system using virtual slides. Diagn Pathol. 2012;7(1):177. doi:10.1186/1746-1596-7-177.
6. Singh R, Hanna M, Parwani A, Pantanowitz L, Punjabi V. Smartphone applications: a contemporary resource for dermatopathology. J Pathol Inform. 2015;6(1):44. doi:10.4103/2153-3539.161612.
7. Kumar V, Abbas A, Fausto N, Aster J. Robbins and cotran pathologic basis of disease. 8th ed. Philadelphia: Saunders; 2010.
8. Cdc.gov. CDC – skin cancer statistics. 2015. Available at: http://www.cdc.gov/cancer/skin/statistics/. Accessed 5 Oct 2015.

9. Brash D, Rudolph J, Simon J, et al. A role for sunlight in skin cancer: UV-induced p53 mutations in squamous cell carcinoma. Proc Natl Acad Sci. 1991;88(22):10124–8. doi:10.1073/pnas.88.22.10124.
10. De Zwaan S, Haass N. Genetics of basal cell carcinoma. Australas J Dermatol. 2009;51(2):81–92. doi:10.1111/j.1440-0960.2009.00579.x.
11. Maloney M. Histology of basal cell carcinoma. Clin Dermatol. 1995;13(6):545–9. doi:10.1016/0738-081x(95)00063-l.
12. Wong C, Strange R, Lear J. Basal cell carcinoma. BMJ. 2003;327:794–8.
13. Aad.org. Skin cancer | aad.org. 2015. Available at: https://www.aad.org/media-resources/stats-and-facts/conditions/skin-cancer. Accessed 5 Oct 2015.
14. Seer.cancer.gov. Melanoma of the Skin – SEER Stat Fact Sheets. 2015. Available at: http://seer.cancer.gov/statfacts/html/melan.html. Accessed 5 Oct 2015.
15. Nelson A, Tsao H. Melanoma and genetics. Clin Dermatol. 2009;27(1):46–52. doi:10.1016/j.clindermatol.2008.09.005.
16. Hosler G, Murphy K. Molecular diagnostics for dermatology. New York: Springer; 2014.
17. Zhang J, Tong H, Fu X, et al. Molecular characterization of NF1 and neurofibromatosis type 1 genotype-phenotype correlations in a Chinese population. Sci Rep. 2015;5:11291. doi:10.1038/srep11291.
18. Tee A, Manning B, Roux P, Cantley L, Blenis J. Tuberous sclerosis complex gene products, tuberin and hamartin, control mTOR signaling by acting as a GTPase-activating protein complex toward Rheb. Curr Biol. 2003;13(15):1259–68. doi:10.1016/s0960-9822(03)00506-2.
19. Lehmann A. The xeroderma pigmentosum group D (XPD) gene: one gene, two functions, three diseases. Genes Dev. 2001;15(1):15–23. doi:10.1101/gad.859501.
20. Genetics Home Reference. Xeroderma pigmentosum. 2015. Available at: http://ghr.nlm.nih.gov/condition/xeroderma-pigmentosum. Accessed 12 Oct 2015.
21. Halpern J, Hopping B, Brostoff J. Photosensitivity, corneal scarring and developmental delay: Xeroderma Pigmentosum in a tropical country. Cases J. 2008;1(1):254.
22. Tang J, Mackay-Wiggan J, Aszterbaum M, et al. Inhibiting the hedgehog pathway in patients with the basal-cell nevus syndrome. N Engl J Med. 2012;366(23):2180–8. doi:10.1056/nejmoa1113538.
23. Devakumar D, Birch M, Osrin D, Sondorp E, Wells J. The intergenerational effects of war on the health of children. BMC Med. 2014;12:57. doi: 10.1186/1741-7015-12-57.
24. Wong LJ, Wong H, Liu A. Intergenerational transmission of pathogenic heteroplasmic mitochondrial DNA. Genet Med. 2002;4(2):78–83.
25. Jarvis WK, Boniface M, Jane Wardle D. The intergenerational transmission of thinness. J Arch Pediatr Adolesc Med. 2011;165(10):900–5.
26. Norman R. The future direction of dermatologic therapy. Skin Aging. 2005;47:32–4.
27. Norman R. The blue man and other stories of the skin. Los Angeles: University of California Press; 2014.

Chapter 5
The Evolution of Human Skin and the Thousands of Species It Sustains, with Ten Hypothesis of Relevance to Doctors

Robert R. Dunn

Abstract The entire skin is covered in microscopic life. The composition of this life—which species are present—has great importance for many aspects of dermatology. Little about this composition makes sense, except in light of evolution.

Keywords Armpits • Bacteria • Belly buttons • Genitals • Wafting

Our skin is what we most immediately perceive of each other. It is the largest human organ [1, 2] and the one through which our bodies meet the world and all of its delights and assaults. It is also, to an extraordinary extent, misunderstood. Here I discuss the key moments in our evolutionary history that are likely to have shaped our skin relative to that of other primates and mammals. I then offer a half dozen hypothesis as to the adaptive role of our skin and the species that live on. In each case, considering our skin in light of evolution and ecology fundamentally alters (or, in the more speculative cases, has the potential to alter) our understanding of its problems and their treatment.

The Ancient History of the Skin

The surface of the body is an ancient feature of all animals. In all animals it serves to protect the body. In a small subset of animals this protection is due primarily to the physical and chemical features of the surface itself. In termites, for example, the

R.R. Dunn, PhD
Department of Applied Ecology and Keck Center for Behavioral Biology, North Carolina State University, Raleigh, NC 27607, USA

Center for Macroecology, Evolution and Climate, Natural History Museum of Denmark, University of Copenhagen, Copenhagen DK-2100, Denmark
e-mail: rrdunn@ncsu.edu

R.A. Norman (ed.), *Personalized, Evolutionary, and Ecological Dermatology*,
DOI 10.1007/978-3-319-41088-3_5

termite integument has evolved a smooth, surface that makes it easy for the termites to groom off pathogens. If one puts an individual fungal spore on the body of a termite, that termite's brothers and sisters will groom the spore off, ingesting it and, in doing so, preventing it from making its way into the bodies of its kin. The termite's integument evolved in such a way as to make it easy for termites to keep their outer surfaces sterile (their inner surfaces, on the other hand, abound with microbes on which they depend. Most medicine has proceeded, across the last hundred years, as though something similar is true for humans and other vertebrates, as though the skins of vertebrates, like the exoskeletons of termites, were sterile but for the occasional arrival of a pathogen. This is not the case.

In many, perhaps most, animals, including all mammal and bird species studied to date, the outer layer of the body is more complex. In such species, it is impossible to prevent organisms from colonizing the body and so animals have instead evolved outer coverings and glands that help to favor beneficial organisms by producing the habitats and food they prefer and disfavor problematic organisms through the production of selective antimicrobial compounds [3]. In such species (including humans) the outer surface is not smooth and sterile but instead colonized by a dense layer of microbes, microbes actively fed and specifically housed by the body. The microbes on the human body are a great extent predictable as a function of the biology of the skin and its glands [4–6], and hence best viewed as an ecosystem engineered by the skin (and genes) and, hence, an ecosystem under the influence of natural selection.[1] In healthy individuals this ecosystem includes hundreds, if not thousands, of kinds of bacteria,[2] viruses that attack those bacteria, archaea, protists and even animals such as mites.

The beneficial microbes living on the skin have can play multiple roles.[3] They are the first line of defense against pathogens [7, 8]. Most pathogens never encounter

[1] We tend to think of beavers as ecosystem engineers in as much as their behaviors, which are encoded by their genes, lead them to build damns and lodges. These behaviors and the genes that underlie them are under natural selection such that natural selection can favor one lodge type over another via its effects on genes that influence behavior. In the same way, our bodies engineer the ecosystem that lives on them and natural selection can influence this ecosystem through its effects on our skin, its glands and the compounds produces in those glands. Our engineered skin ecosystem, in short, evolves.

[2] Although this diversity is great, it is in some ways deceptive. Many species of bacteria, for example, are found on the skin, but these species derive disproportionately from just a handful of the bacterial phyla found in any pinch of soil. Best represented are the phyla Actinobacteria, Firmicutes, Proteobacteria and Bacteroidetes. Then within these phyla a few genera are disproportionately important, particularly *Corynebacterium*, *Staphylococcus*, *Propionibacterium*, and *Streptococcus*.

[3] Of note, beneficial is a term with some baggage. Mutualisms such as those described here are relationships in which organisms of two different species both benefit from each other's presence. However, mutualism is always a term reflecting the net condition. A beneficial microbe might have some costs, so long as its net effect is benefit. Similarly, the costs and benefits of any particular microbial species to human or other hosts are conditional. They depend on circumstances. A species that was beneficial 12,000 years ago to humans, might not be today. By the same token, a species that was not historically beneficial might be beneficial in light of our modern diets and lifestyles. In as much as human bodies (and their underlying genes) evolve relatively slowly this has the potential to lead to mismatches between the microbes our bodies favor and those that benefit us.

mammal immune systems; they instead first encounter the microbes living on mammal fur and skin, microbes with the ability to kill pathogens, whether through the production of antimicrobials (to which they themselves are resistant) or through other means of competition. In other words, the microbes on the skin are a defensive layer. Skin microbes also aid in the development of the immune systems. Unlike, for example, the heart, the immune system does not develop in isolation, it develops in interaction with skin and gut microbes. Many immune disorders now seem to relate to problems during this development [9–11].

Beneficial skin microbes are also used by mammals in finding mates. Skin microbes produce volatile (airborne) compounds during metabolism. Many mammals use these compounds as pheromones. Pheromone signals are then altered through changes in what the body feeds skin and gland microbes (In humans, the microbe food is altered in response to stress, and sexual activity, for instance). What do skin microbe volatiles signal? We are only beginning to learn. Based on insights from ecology and evolution, however, it seems likely that these volatiles provide signals of the genetic background of the host (which immune genes the host has, for example). In as much as it is costly for the host to feed the microbes on the skin, these volatiles might also be an honest signal of host health; it is, one might speculate, only possible to feed an abundance of skin microbes and their bouquet if well fed. Odors also provide a signal of group membership; hyenas recognize those individuals who are part of their group based on the odors of their bacteria [12]. Finally, it has long been known that individual hosts infected by pathogens produce unique odors. The absence of these pathogen odors and the presence of the odor of healthy microbes might also be a signal of health. It is interesting in this regard to note that the ability of some cats and dogs to identify humans who are sick may relate to the ability of the cats and dogs themselves to identify other cats and dogs that are sick so as to avoid mating with them.

Finally, in as much as this layer of life has been present on mammals and other vertebrates for hundreds of millions of years, those organisms that seek out mammals as food use them to find those mammals. In doing so, they are conducting a sort of ecological espionage, honing in on signals meant for potential mates, or accidental signals of the processes being carried out by beneficial microbes. Mosquitoes, for instance, find mammal hosts by flying up the rivers of CO_2 that flow out of their mouths, but appear to choose which mammal to bite based on the smell of the volatile compounds produced by skin microbes. The odor of some microbes attracts mosquitoes; the odors of others repel them [13, 14]. The presence of these repellent microbes may then be a benefit in terms of deterrence of mosquitoes.

In short, for hundreds of millions of years the skin has really been three things, the skin itself, the organisms living on the skin, and the glands of the skin, a key role of which is to feed and favor some organisms relative to others. If we think about the skin in this light, and as ecosystem that has evolved in response to natural selection, many new hypotheses emerge as to the function of strange attributes of mammal skin in general and human skin as specific case, for example, the problem of stinky feet.

Hypothesis 1: Stinky foot bacteria are beneficial I do not need to tell you that human feet can be stinky. In this, we are not unique. Dog feet have a characteristic odor, as do those of cats and pigs. In each case, this characteristic odor is produced by a particular mélange of bacteria. In humans, two dominant odor producers are *Staphylococcus epidermidis* and *Bacillus subtilis*. It is *Bacillus subtilis* ("subtilis" being a misnomer on par with, for example, Greenland) that can lead feet to smell like a mix between, say, dead squirrel and rotten fish. The standard approach to thinking about these odors, to the extent anyone wants to mention them at all, is to ponder how to get rid of them. Evolutionary thinking, however, begs a different question. It begs us to ask why feet stink in the first place.

Until very recently most humans walked barefoot. When walking barefoot humans, like most mammals, we are very susceptible to foot injuries (cuts and scrapes) that could become infected, particularly by fungi. Fungal infections are more problematic for mammals in those parts of the body where circulation is poor, which include the feet. Given that this is the case, it would be adaptive if human foot skin had evolved to favor bacteria that produce antifungal compounds.

It may be that the unique bacteria of modern feet (including the dominance *Bacillus subtilis*) are due to the use of shoes and socks (I know of no studies of the foot bacteria of individuals who do not wear shoes). But for a moment, let's assume that this is not the case. Could the body conceivably have a way to favor specific bacteria on feet? And if so, why?

We know that the body produces large amounts of sweat through the feet (far more than is necessary for cooling, and why cool the feet anyway?). This sweat is enriched for leucine relative to other parts of the body [15] an expensive amino acid. *Bacillus subtilis* thrives on leucine. It is in metabolizing leucine that *B. subtilis* produces isoflavic acid the compound characteristic of the smell of stinky feet [16]. *Bacillus subtilis* also produces antifungals, antifungals that, for instance, are capable, at least in the lab of killing several fungi often found as pathogens on feet [17]. In other words, our feet may have evolved to produce lots of sweat, with leucine, to feed specific bacteria that kill fungi that reduce our risk of foot infection.

The idea that our bodies actively feed specific foot bacteria as a defense against fungal pathogens needs to be tested. But if right it has important implications particularly for individuals, such as those who are immune-compromised or diabetic, namely that any behaviors that make bacteria with metabolic abilities similar to *Bacillus subtilis* less abundant are likely to increase our risk of foot infections.

Hypothesis 2: The initial composition of microbes on the skin influences the likelihood and rate of wound healing This is a simple idea, so simple that one might imagine it has been very well-studied. A variety of studies have begun to link the abundance of specific microbes on the skin to diseases states. Psoriasis lesions, for example, have a relatively greater abundance of Firmicutes and relatively fewer Actinobacteria and Proteobacteria than does health skin [18]. Patients with atopic dermatitis tend to have a lower diversity of skin microbes than do individuals with healthy skin; their skin is dominated by species of *Staphylococcus* [19]. It is almost inevitably true that the precise composition of microbes on the skin where a wound occurs is likely to influence the healing of a wound. This doesn't seem like an Earth shattering statement, but as far as I know no clinicians actively measure the composition of skin microbes before considering treatment of wounds and infections. At most individual microbe taxa (e.g., specific pathogens) are searched for. We know that wound healing varies greatly among humans, among human body parts, and between humans and other mammals. This variation must be in part due to variation in the initial composition of microbes.

Hypothesis 3 No infection of a mammal, ever, on Earth, has ever been due to just a single species of pathogen. Every infection will always involve both the pathogen or pathogens and all of the commensal species with which it is interacting. Most infections likely represent the actions and chemical compounds due to tens if not hundreds of species. Again, this seems obvious. Again, if it is true it calls for different and new approaches to surgical incisions, surgeries, wounds and infections.

More ancient history of the skin, including face mites Face mites (*Demodex spp.)* appear to have evolved with the origin of mammals [20]. They live inside hair follicles and glands. Very few species of mammals have been studied for their *Demodex* face mites; yet it is likely that all mammals possess one or probably more often more than one species found nowhere else (and given that these mites are host specific, this would mean that there might be as many as 10,000 *Demodex* species, two per mammal species, even though only a few tens are so far named). Humans are host to two named species of face mites, *Demodex folliculorum* and *Demodex brevis*, and based on our research, additional as of yet named species [21, 22]. All adult humans have these mites in the follicles on their faces but also elsewhere on the body. These mites become more abundant in conditions of mange, and also in humans with rosacea. In neither case, however, do the mites appear to cause these diseases (though they are clearly part of the story). The average human host, like the average mammal host more generally is likely to host tens of thousands, but perhaps even hundreds of thousands of individual mites on his or her body. These mites and their abundance have been a dependable presence with which mammal bodies have coevolved for more than a 100 million years. In light of the ancient biology of these mites, I offer an additional hypothesis.

Hypothesis 4 Counterintuitively, *Demodex* face mites could be used cure rosacea. Rosacea is a common immune-related problem of the skin. It seems likely that one could devise a clinical treatment with face mites that could actually help to treat rosacea. Given the abundance of face mites on humans, that we do not generate an immune response to these mites most of the time means they are producing, almost certainly, immunosuppressants. If we could harness these immunosuppressants we might use them in treating rosacea. An alternate approach would be to manipulate the composition of bacteria living in face mites. It has been suggested that while face mites themselves do not cause rosacea, that perhaps particular bacteria associated with the mites do. If this were the case, one could imagine manipulations of the microbiomes of face mites in ways that remedy rosacea. In as much as all adults, regardless of their hygiene behavior, appear to have face mites, the idea of treating skin disorders through manipulation of mite composition is perhaps less radical than it initially seems.

Ape Skin

Primates in general, when compared to other mammals, seem to be particularly rich in glands. If we take the function of these glands to primarily be to alter microbial composition of the skin, then this diversity and abundance of glands represents a rich arena for future studies likely to alter our understanding of what it is to be a primate. Some of these glands, however, we know a little more about, among them a set that are more common in apes (gorillas, monkeys, chimpanzees, bonobos, humans) than in other primates, the apocrine glands. Apocrine glands are concentrated in the armpits, around the nipples, in the belly button and perianal and genital regions. They produce compounds that feed a subset of slow growing microbes, including species of *Corynebacterium*. As a result of the food given to *Corynebacterium* species by apocrine glands, these bacteria and their relatives are far more abundant in apes than in other primates [23]. *Corynebacterium* bacteria seems likely to be fed by ape bodies because they offer some value to the apes [24, 25].

Hypothesis 5 The increased investment in apocrine glands, their products and microbes in apes is likely to have been due to changes in the need for one of the roles of such microbes, whether as a pheromone, in pathogen defense, or in deterrence of mosquito vectors of pathogens. This possibility has gone totally unexplored. By the same token, the differences in the apocrine glands and their bacteria among ape species are likely to reflect differences in the mating biology, pathogen and vector risk of these primates.

Hypothesis 6: Apocrine bacteria help to defend us against infection Apocrine glands are larger and more dense and differently distributed in humans than in other apes and in other apes than in primates more generally [26–29], as would be expected if these glands had been evolving recently in response to selection to play a more rather than less important role.[4] These glands are found in the armpits, but also in other regions where bacterial (rather than fungal) infections are common. These include the belly button, where infection after birth can be deadly, the perianal and vaginal regions. We also know that under stress that the microbes in the apocrine glands are fed more by our bodies, become more abundant and secrete more extracellular compounds. I hypothesize that the apocrine glands play the role, in part, of preventing infection in wounds and other openings to the body cavity. In line with this prediction I recently received a call from a doctor who noted that in his

[4] In addition, key features of the cell biology of human skin, including the sugars associated with cells, are also different from those in other apes in ways that seem likely to be of most consequence to microbes [33].

practice that he had dramatically reduced his rate of surgical infection through laparoscopic surgery. This is what would be expected if the bacteria being fed by the apocrine glands in the belly button help to prevent infection.

Early Hominid Skin

The skin is an unusual organ in many regards, not least of which because the skin of humans differs in many ways from that of our closest living relatives. In short, we are naked. They are furry. Our bodies are not, of course, totally naked (nor are all other mammals totally furry. See, for example, naked mole rats). We have diminutive hairs all over our bodies. But these hairs are too small to be of functional consequence. Too small to keep warm or protect us from the sun [30]. A relatively large literature has considered the loss of hair from human skin, our "nakedness," in no small part because this nakedness predisposes us to many of the most common skin problems, including skin cancers. It makes wounds more likely, something I have noticed on the top of my head since losing one of those few bits of hair humans maintain (or that many humans do anyway). It is also this nakedness that required our ancestors, in moving into cold environments, to invent clothes. One might also contend that our views of nudity, body art and style all also relate in one way or another to our naked condition. If we were covered in yak-like fur, nude beaches would be less titillating (and more sweaty). A relatively large literature now considers this loss of fur. Among the most plausible explanations for it relates to the pathogens vectored by ectoparasites.

Hypothesis 7 One body of work suggests that the skin of humans is relatively naked due to the influence of ectoparasites. In being hairless humans have escaped to a great extent high densities of lice, fleas, some mites and other arthropods that live in the fur. To remove a louse from your skin you need only squish it and wash your clothes. No such luxury exists for your cat. It is hypothesized that the genes of any of our ancestors who were less hairy and louse-bitten were favored because many arthropods transmit pathogens. Those of our ancestors with less hair may have been less likely to die of the infections ectoparasites transmit.

Hypothesis 8 Conversely, *hairier individuals are almost certainly host to different organisms (be they multi- or single-celled) and, as a result, will have different risks associated with medical interventions.*

More, Early Human Skin

In addition to the risk to early humans posed by vector born pathogens, early humans also began to face many new pathogens more generally. That this is the case is beyond debate. Modern humans are now host to more than 200 pathogen species, whereas fewer than a 100 infect gorillas and chimpanzees (for example). As a result of this shift, we know many shifts in human genes, particularly those associated with immune systems. It is likely that skin biology, and skin microbiology in particular, also changed in response to the transition to environments in which pathogens were more common. One can imagine many changes. I'll just offer one, a change related to the increase in the risk of vector-borne diseases in early human settlements.

Hypothesis 9: In malarial regions human skin is more likely to favor microbes that are less attractive to malaria mosquitoes Once vector-borne pathogens became prevalent in human societies strong selective pressures would have favored individual human lineages with skin that was less attractive to vectors. These lineages would have been favored disproportionately in those regions where malaria has been common the longest.

Our Modern Skin

Our modern skin differs from that of other apes because of our loss of fur and unique glands, but it also differs from that of humans living just a few 100 years ago. Hygiene has changed dramatically in the last 200 years. Based on historical sources (e.g., gross and detailed stories of the washing habits of kings) and studies of non-human primates, it seems as though until relatively recently that the washing of human bodies was relatively rare, that feces and fecal microbes could often be found on the body, and that slow growing microbes could have grown with little interruption so long as they could compete with other microbes [31, 32].

Even before the advent of hygiene products such as antiperspirants and body sprays modern hygiene led the slow growing microbes on the body to be disturbed with high frequency. It also washed fecal microbes from the skin and hair. These changes have been hugely beneficial to public health, but in as much as they are changes relative to the conditions in which our bodies evolved over the last 300 million years (or more), they are probably not without unintended consequences. In addition, however, to these changes we now know that antiperspirants have a large effect on skin microbes. They, quite predictably, disfavor the microbes fed by our apocrine glands, and favor fast growing species. The microbes we now think of as the medically normal inhabitants of the skin (such as *Staphylococcus*) are composed almost exclusively of those favored by the use of antiperspirants and, before that, likely by public health in general [31, 32].

Hypothesis 10: Antiperspirant use makes our skin more susceptible to infection Our armpits contain many apocrine glands that appear to have evolved to feed *Corynebateria* species and their relatives. Antiperspirants work by closing down the function of apocrine glands. This leads *Corynebacteria* species to become less abundant. This in turn favors a high diversity of relatively unusual bacteria. Those bacteria include *Staphylococcus* bacteria, including, I will speculate, the subset of fast-growing Staphylococcus most likely to be pathogenic.

Conclusions

We still know relatively little about the evolution of human skin and the species associated with it. No comprehensive survey has yet considered the skin in full. We do not know, for example, how many and which animal species live on the skin. It is likely that many more animal species, in addition to *Demodex* mites, are common even on healthy humans. A second necessity is more thorough study of the skin and skin biology of non-human primates and other mammals. The literature, for example, on the evolution of skin glands of primates has scarcely been improved on in the last 50 years. A third necessity is an understanding of the genetics of these changes. Finally, and most importantly, this collective understanding must be brought to bear on modern medicine. We still do medicine as though our bodies were sterile vessels, sterile termite-like bodies on which the occasional pathogen lands. Until this perspective changes, until we recognize the richness on our skin and its consequences, we will continue to make clinical choices that leave patients unhappy, sick and, in many cases, dead.

References

1. Leider M, Buncke CM. Physical dimensions of the skin: determination of the specific gravity of skin, hair, and nail. AMA Arch Dermatol Syphilol. 1954;69(5):563–9.
2. Goldsmith LA. My organ is bigger than your organ. Arch Dermatol. 1990;126(3):301–2.
3. Peschel A, Jack RW, Otto M, et al. *Staphylococcus aureus* resistance to human defensins and evasion of neutrophil killing via the novel virulence factor MprF is based on modification of membrane lipids with l-lysine. J Exp Med. 2001;193:1067–76.
4. Grice EA, Kong HH, Conlan S, Deming CB, Davis J, Young AC, et al. Topographical and temporal diversity of the human skin microbiome. Science. 2009;324(5931):1190–2.
5. Hulcr J, Latimer AM, Henley JB, Rountree NR, Fierer N, Lucky A, et al. A jungle in there: bacteria in belly buttons are highly diverse, but predictable. PLoS One. 2012;7(11):e47712.
6. Kong HH. Skin microbiome: genomics-based insights into the diversity and role of skin microbes. Trends Mol Med. 2011;17(6):320–8.
7. Christensen G, Brüggemann H. Bacterial skin commensals and their role as host guardians. Benef Microbes. 2014;5(2):201–15.
8. Park B, Iwase T, Liu GY. Intranasal application of *S. epidermidis* prevents colonization by methicillin-resistant *Staphylococcus aureus* in mice. PLoS One. 2011;6(10):e25880.
9. Belkaid Y, Segre JA. Dialogue between skin microbiota and immunity. Science. 2014;346(6212):954–9.
10. Tlaskalová-Hogenová H, Štěpánková R, Hudcovic T, Tučková L, Cukrowska B, Lodinová-Žádníková R, et al. Commensal bacteria (normal microflora), mucosal immunity and chronic inflammatory and autoimmune diseases. Immunol Lett. 2004;93(2):97–108.
11. Grice EA, Segre JA. The skin microbiome. Nat Rev Microbiol. 2011;9(4):244–53.
12. Theis KR, Schmidt TM, Holekamp KE. Evidence for a bacterial mechanism for group-specific social odors among hyenas. Sci Rep. 2012;2:615.
13. Verhulst NO, Beijleveld H, Knols BG, Takken W, Schraa G, Bouwmeester HJ, et al. Cultured skin microbiota attracts malaria mosquitoes. Malar J. 2009;8(1):302.
14. Verhulst NO, Qiu YT, Beijleveld H, Maliepaard C, Knights D, Schulz S, et al. Composition of human skin microbiota affects attractiveness to malaria mosquitoes. PLoS One. 2011;6(12):e28991.

15. Hadorn B, Hanimann F, Anders P, Curtius HC, Halverson R. Free amino-acids in human sweat from different parts of the body. Nature (Lond). 1967;215:416.
16. Ara K, et al. Foot odor due to microbial metabolism and its control. Can J Microbiol. 2006;52:357–64.
17. Landy MWGH, Roseman SB, Colio LG. Bacillomycin, an antibiotic from *Bacillus subtilis* active against pathogenic fungi. Proc Soc Exp Biol Med. 1948;67:539–41.
18. Gao Z, Tseng CH, Strober BE, Pei Z, Blaser MJ. Substantial alterations of the cutaneous bacterial biota in psoriatic lesions. PLoS One. 2008;3:e2719.
19. Kong HH, Oh J, Deming C, Conlan S, Grice EA, Beatson MA, Nomicos E, Polley EC, Komarow HD, Program NCS, Murray PR, Turner ML, Segre JA. Temporal shifts in the skin microbiome associated with disease flares and treatment in children with atopic dermatitis. Genome Res. 2012;22:850–9.
20. Palopoli MF, et al. Complete mitochondrial genomes of the human follicle mites Demodex brevis and D. folliculorum: novel gene arrangement, truncated tRNA genes, and ancient divergence between species. BMC Genomics. 2014;15(1):1124.
21. Thoemmes MS, et al. Ubiquity and diversity of human-associated Demodex mites. PLoS One. 2014;9:e106265.
22. Palopoli MF, et al. Global divergence of the human follicle mite Demodex folliculorum: persistent associations between host ancestry and mite lineages. Proc Natl Acad Sci. 2015;112:15958–63.
23. Council SE, Savage AM, Urban JM, et al. Diversity and evolution of the primate skin microbiome. Proc Biol Sci. 2016;283(1822):pii: 20152586.
24. James AG, Austin CJ, Cox DS, Taylor D, Calvert R. Microbiological and biochemical origins of human axillary odour. FEMS Microbiol Ecol. 2013;83(3):527–40.
25. Leyden JJ, McGinley KJ, Hölzle E, Labows JN, Kligman AM. The microbiology of the human axilla and its relationship to axillary odor. J Invest Dermatol. 1981;77(5):413–6.
26. Montagna W. The evolution of human skin. J Hum Evol. 1985;14(1):3–22.
27. Ellis RA, Montagna W. The skin of primates. VI. The skin of the gorilla (*Gorilla gorilla*). Am J Phys Anthropol. 1962;20(2):79–93.
28. Prüfer K, Munch K, Hellmann I, Akagi K, Miller JR, Walenz B, et al. The bonobo genome compared with the chimpanzee and human genomes. Nature. 2012;486(7404):527–31.
29. Folk Jr GE, Semken Jr A. The evolution of sweat glands. Int J Biometeorol. 1991;35(3):180–6.
30. Kushlan JA. The evolution of hairlessness in man. Am Nat. 1980;116:727–9.
31. Shelley WB, Hurley HJ, Nichols AC. Axillary odor: experimental study of the role of bacteria, apocrine sweat, and deodorants. AMA Arch Dermatol Syphilol. 1953;68(4):430–46.
32. Urban J, Fergus DJ, Savage AM, Ehlers M, Menninger HL, Dunn RR, Horvath JE. The effect of habitual and experimental antiperspirant and deodorant product use on the armpit microbiome. Peer J. 2016;4:e1605. https://doi.org/10.7717/peerj.1605.
33. Nguyen DH, Hurtado-Ziola N, Gagneux P, Varki A. Loss of Siglec expression on T lymphocytes during human evolution. Proc Natl Acad Sci U S A. 2006;103(20):7765–70.

Chapter 6
What's New in Dermatopathology?

Jeff Collins, Pam Kittipongdaja, and Michael Morgan

Abstract DNA microarrays were developed in the mid 1990s and are an efficient tool that can take a snapshot of a cells active expressed DNA. By allowing fast and inexpensive analysis, microarrays have exploded in use. They work by fixing a short segment of cDNA or segment of oligonucleotides called a probe, to a silicon or glass backing. The probes are exposed to tissue extracted nucleic acids and if present will bind to the probe causing fluorescence. A single microarray chip the length of a matchstick can fit tens of thousands of probes at relatively low cost providing significant advantage over other techniques.

Keywords Dermatopathology • Diagnostic • Molecular • Teledermatopathology • Immunohistochemistry • Infectious disease

Diagnostic Molecular Dermatopathology

DNA microarrays were developed in the mid 1990s and are an efficient tool that can take a snapshot of a cells active expressed DNA [1]. By allowing fast and inexpensive analysis, microarrays have exploded in use. They work by fixing a short segment of cDNA or segment of oligonucleotides called a probe, to a silicon or glass backing. The probes are exposed to tissue extracted nucleic acids and if present will bind to the probe causing fluorescence. A single microarray chip the length of a

J. Collins, DO
Advanced Dermatology and Cosmetic Surgery, Maitland, FL, USA

P. Kittipongdaja, DO
Advanced Dermatology and Cosmetic Surgery, University of South Florida Morsani College of Medicine, Tampa, FL, USA

M. Morgan, MD, PhD (✉)
Dermatology and Cosmetic Surgery, Michigan State University College of Osteopathic Medicine, East Lansing, MI, USA

University of South Florida Morsani College of Medicine, Tampa, FL, USA
e-mail: mbkmmorgan@aol.com

R.A. Norman (ed.), *Personalized, Evolutionary, and Ecological Dermatology*, DOI 10.1007/978-3-319-41088-3_6

matchstick can fit tens of thousands of probes at relatively low cost providing significant advantage over other techniques [2].

For the most part all of our cells contain our full genome, however it is selectively expressed. Each cell type is rendered unique by the specific set of genes that are active. A microarray chip can provide snapshot information on what genes and subsequent translated proteins the cell is currently expressing, that is its “transcriptional profile” [3]. By running a microarray on both healthy skin and cancer, one can compare the pattern of proteins- yielding clues as to what might be overexpressed or suppressed in a malignant cell. Researchers can extrapolate this to almost any disease state, comparing the transcriptional profile of healthy skin side by side to that of atopic dermatitis, psoriasis and skin aging [4].

Microarrays and future genetic sequencing will be used to change the landscape of personalized medicine. Because of its accessibility, skin and dermatology has been at the forefront of microarray use. They have provided large amounts of data requiring heavy computer and technology use- driving the formation of “skinomics” [3]. To run side by side microarrays, a biopsy isn’t even needed to acquire the genetic material. Non-invasive and simple tape stripping can get enough nucleic material to run a microarray [5]. In the future, “skinomics” will power pan scanning of tumor specimens for mutations. The expanded list of mutations will open opportunities for development of additional targeted therapies. In addition to H&E, a pathology report of the future might come with a transcriptional profile printout and the corresponding diagnoses that have a similar profile. Skinomics and DNA studies will also be able to shed light on currently ambiguous subjects like the grading and management of dysplastic nevi. The pathology report of the future for a dysplastic nevus will show the genetic fingerprint and compare that to melanoma [6]. This will better enable clinicians to decipher which truly need excision and which can be monitored. Using combination of tape stripping and microarrays to determine genetic profile, melanoma can already be diagnosed without a biopsy [7]. Pathology specimens of the future may not be in a formalin bottle but rather a piece of tape.

The current cost per amount of data obtained, widespread adaptability, and efficiency gives microarrays a significant edge for the near future. However as DNA&RNA sequencing declines in cost it will likely supplant microarrays. RNA-seq is a powerful tool to decipher a transcriptional profile far beyond the limitations of microarrays, including an unprecedented capability to discover novel genes, alternative transcript variants, chimeric transcripts, and expressed sequence variants as well as allele-specific expression [8]. Both the cost and data heavy processing are current barriers to sequencing technology. For the present time microarray’s are the most cost effective way to obtain a genetic and a transcriptional profile. In the future, DNA microarrays and skinomics will be available for bedside use, enabling the clinician to get enhanced understanding of the healthy and pathological processes in skin, including neoplasms, inflammatory diseases, genodermatoses, wound healing, cosmetic dermatology etc.

Among the many practical and current adaptations of DNA nucleotide technology is testing for oncogene expression in the potentially deadly cutaneous disease-melanoma. BRAF was discovered in 2002 and already has FDA approved targeted therapy on the market [9]. It has spawned a cascade of research in melanoma mutations, all driven by molecular diagnostics. A 2015 study genetically scanned 699 melanomas and the most common mutations were BRAFV600 (36 %), NRAS (21 %), TP53 (16 %), BRAFNon-V600 (6 %), and KIT (4 %) [10]. This is a slight departure from the pioneering BRAF study in 2002 that report BRAF mutations at 66 % [9].

Three functional RAF proteins exist in humans, ARAF, BRAF, and CRAF. Among them, BRAF has the highest basal kinase activity, and is the most potent activator of the MAPK pathway. The mutation results in a substitution of glutamic acid for valine at position 600, which is designated as V600E. This mutation turns BRAF into an potent oncogene and is reported to have 10 times more kinase activity than its normal counterpart [9]. Less common V600 substitutions constitute about 12 % of BRAF mutations and consist of V600K as well as V600D. Targeted anti BRAF therapy has already been synergistically combined with anti MEK therapies to block both the main and alternative pathways and has shown promising clinical outcome.

Currently the PCR based COBAS 4800 BRAF V600 Mutation Test- is the superior method to test BRAF. It can identify at least 96 % of mutations across all specimen types with 5 % mutant alleles at a DNA input of 125 ng, an amount readily obtained from one 5-μm section of formalin-fixed paraffin-embedded tissue [11, 12]. The test is highly reproducible (98.8 %) and has been shown to be more accurate than direct sequencing [11]. Failures in melanoma molecular diagnostics are normally the result of poor fixation of pathological specimens, the age of the sample and high levels of pigmentation.

A small number of overall melanomas about 4–10 % but relative high percentage of mucosal, and acral melanomas (40 %), also have changes in the *C-KIT* gene [13]. This encodes for a tyrosine kinase receptor and can be targeted by tyrosine kinase inhibitors like imatinib. These drugs have been very effective in other cancers with the same mutation. Early clinical trials were very disappointing but were finalized before KIT mutations were well known in melanoma and didn't screen for them [14]. When selecting for mutations affecting the recurrent hot spots or with a mutant/wild-type allelic ratio of >1, the response rate was 40 % [14]. These findings indicate that an accurate identification of *KIT* mutation is both practical and necessary to select patients who may benefit from imatinib treatment. Newer-generation KIT inhibitors, such as dasatinib, nilotinib and masitinib have shown more efficacy than imatinib but still will not likely be used as monotherapy. Much like vemurafenib (BRAF) is combined with trametinib (MEK) we hypothesize that in the future CKIT therapy will be combined dual therapy. At this point KIT inhibitors would most likely be combined with ipilimumab (anti CTLA-4) or nivolumab (anti PD-1) [15].

We hypothesize that in the future melanoma's will be pan scanned for genetic mutations now typically only available in a research setting. It is likely that a diagnostic report for melanoma will not only have the synoptic parameters of breslow depth, ulceration and mitotic rate but the status of BFAF, KIT plus future unknown oncogenes as well as drug susceptibilities for chemotherapy agents. BRAF and cKIT are the only mutations now routinely tested in clinical practice. They are usually only tested when you are considering systemic chemotherapy in advanced melanoma. Future genetic testing of thin stage I and stage II melanomas still will not likely be necessary as very high cure rates are achievable with wide local excision. Mutation targeted treatments are already available for BRAF (vemurafinib), BRAF nonV600E (sorafenib), C-KIT (imatinib), and MEK (trametinib). There are ongoing clinical trials targeting the additional pathways NRAS, PI3k, and AKT, providing additional future therapies.

As staggering advances in scientific basic and translational research have been applied to clinical dermatology, so too have been implemented in the practice of dermatopathology. This portion of the chapter will focus on the current technologies of digital teledermatopathology, and applied immunohistochemistry, technology of DNA microarray, oncogene and prognostic marker validation testing.

Teledermatopathology

Modern advances in communication technology have propelled the use of teledermatopathology for the distant diagnosis of skin specimens. Teledermatopathology has many benefits, apart from allowing timely consultation from a remote location, it can help link rural and underserved communities that lack access to a subspecialty-trained dermatopathologist. In addition, teledermatopathology can save both time and money by eliminating the cost and time associated with sending glass slides [16, 17]. Despite these potential benefits, teledermatopathology is still not used routinely. The major hurdles that prevent its wide adoption are concerns about diagnostic accuracy, the state-to-state variation in licensure requirement and reimbursement [18].

There are three main approaches to transmitting the images: static store and forward system, live real-time transmission, and a hybrid virtual slide systems (VSS). Static store and forward system involves the transfer of individually captured digital images of the histologic slides at varied magnifications subjectively selected by the referring pathologist [19]. These images are then transmitted to a consulting pathologist either by e-mail, File Transfer Protocol connection, or using a specific Web application [19]. This technology is relative simple and less expensive than other methods. Most recently, the technology has evolved from static-image based systems to whole slide scanning. The recent introduction of virtual slide systems (VSS) enables the digitization of whole slides at high resolutions thus enabling the user to view any part of the specimen at any magnification [16]. The VSS images are then stored on the server and made available on the web via an integrated VS client network [19]. Another approach is an attempt to reproduce a live, real-time examination of slides via remotely controlled robotic technology. This technology allows consulting pathologists to examine the entire slide digitally with control over slide movement and magnification. Real-time teledermatopathology is more appealing to most pathologists because it closely resembles the established technique of traditional pathologic examination [19].

Many studies have compared the diagnostic accuracy of static image and whole slide imaging system with that of traditional light microscopy. A recent review of studies conducted between 1997 and 2012 comparing the store and forward technology with traditional light microscopy reveals the diagnostic accuracy of the store and forward method to be similar or inferior to conventional light microscopy [18]. However, with improved technology, later studies have shown better diagnostic accuracy. In terms of licensure, most states require out of state physicians to obtain a full in-state medical license in dermatopathology/pathology in order to practice teledermatopathology. Some states allow alternatives to obtaining a full in-state license and a few states will allow physicians to practice teledermatopathology as long as the diagnoses are made infrequently [18]. Similar to licensing, physician reimbursement is state- and payer-dependent. In all states, teledermatopathology is covered by Medicare with billing similar to those performed by an on-site dermatopathologist [18]. Medicaid and private payers coverage and reimbursement varies. Currently, 15 states explicitly mandate that private payers cover telemedicine services, with another 14 states making proposals to state legislature [18].

Immunohistochemistry of Infectious Disease

Immunohistochemistry (IHC) is a method by which specific target antigens can be detected in formalin-fixed paraffin-embedded tissue and involves the use of monoclonal or polyclonal antibodies. IHC continues to be one of the main adjunctive methods in histopathological diagnosis. It has been shown to be useful in identifying microorganisms that are (1) difficult to detect by routine or special stains, (2) stain poorly, (3) present in low numbers, or (4) noncultivable [20].

IHC can be quite useful in herpes virus detection and identification. Immunoperoxidase stains specific for HSV-1, HSV-2, AND VZV are available commercially [21]. The intensity of staining varies between cells depending on the type of infection. In the case of atypical cutaneous infection, IHC can be quite useful. For example, IHC was able to identify HSV infection in 5 bedridden geriatric patients (type I in 3 and type II in 2) with genital ulcers, when histology was suggestive of HSV infection in only 2 of the 5 patients [22]. Another study showed that the sensitivity and specificity of IHC were comparable with in situ hybridization (ISH) in diagnosing HSV [23]. Similarly, IHC has also been shown to exhibit higher specificity and sensitivity than standard microscopic assessments in diagnosing varicella zoster virus (VZV) infection through detection of VZV ORF63 encoded protein (IE63) and VZV late protein GE on both smears and formalin-fixed paraffin-embedded skin sections [24]. Human herpes virus 8 (HHV-8) is also much easier to detect using commercially available monoclonal antibody against the c-terminus of the latent nuclear antigen (LNA-1) [21]. The presence of HHV-8 in the nuclei of proliferating cells in KS lesions may be demonstrated in all its epidemiologic variants and from the earliest phases of the process [21]. LNA-1 has shown to be highly sensitive and specific for the diagnosis of KS and thus allowing its differentiation from its mimickers including angiosarcoma, kaposiform hemangioendothelioma, spindle-cell hemangioma, among others [25, 26].

Treponema pallidum in FFPE tissue sections has classically been identified using silver staining techniques, such as the Levaditi or Warthin–Starry (WS) stains, but immunoperoxidase techniques using polyclonal antibodies against *T. pallidum* improve spirochete visualization with no background staining [21]. In one study, 34 biopsy specimens of patients with primary and secondary syphilis were evaluated. IHC detected spirochetes [27] in 85 % of the biopsies compared to 50 % with Warthin-starry stain [20, 21]. In 2007, Kumar et al. studied the sensitivity and reliability of immunodiagnostic assay for direct detection of *C. trachomatis* [28] infections in endocervical specimens from female patients. For this purpose they developed species-specific monoclonal antibodies that recognized the major outer membrane protein of all serovars of *C. trachomatis*. They compared the reactivity of the developed species-specific monoclonal antibody with the commercially available direct fluorescent antibody test and found that the developed antibody had a higher sensitivity (97.22 %) compared with direct fluorescent antibody and can be used as a reliable method in laboratories for the diagnosis of chlamydial infections.

The use of a continuously increasing number of newly raised and commercially available antibodies for IHC has tremendously broadened IHC applicability for the diagnosis of different types of infections.

References

1. Schena M, Shalon D, Davis RW, Brown PO. Quantitative monitoring of gene expression patterns with a complementary DNA microarray. Science. 1995;270(5235):467–70.
2. Villaseñor-Park J, Ortega-Loayza AG. Microarray technique, analysis, and applications in dermatology. J Invest Dermatol. 2013;133(4):e7.
3. Blumenberg M. SKINOMICS: transcriptional profiling in dermatology and skin biology. Curr Genomics. 2012;13(5):363–8.
4. Rizzo AE, Maibach HI. Personalizing dermatology: the future of genomic expression profiling to individualize dermatologic therapy. J Dermatolog Treat. 2012;23(3):161–7.
5. Wong R, Tran V, Morhenn V, et al. Use of RT-PCR and DNA microarrays to characterize RNA recovered by non-invasive tape harvesting of normal and inflamed skin. J Invest Dermatol. 2004;123(1):159–67.
6. Talantov D, Mazumder A, Yu JX, et al. Novel genes associated with malignant melanoma but not benign melanocytic lesions. Clin Cancer Res. 2005;11(20):7234–42.
7. Wachsman W, Morhenn V, Palmer T, et al. Noninvasive genomic detection of melanoma. Br J Dermatol. 2011;164(4):797–806.
8. Zhang W, Yu Y, Hertwig F, et al. Comparison of RNA-seq and microarray-based models for clinical endpoint prediction. Genome Biol. 2015;16:133.
9. Davies H, Bignell GR, Cox C, et al. Mutations of the BRAF gene in human cancer. Nature. 2002;417(6892):949–54.
10. Siroy AE, Boland GM, Milton DR, et al. Beyond BRAF(V600): clinical mutation panel testing by next-generation sequencing in advanced melanoma. J Invest Dermatol. 2015;135(2):508–15.

11. Halait H, Demartin K, Shah S, et al. Analytical performance of a real-time PCR-based assay for V600 mutations in the BRAF gene, used as the companion diagnostic test for the novel BRAF inhibitor vemurafenib in metastatic melanoma. Diagn Mol Pathol. 2012;21(1):1–8.
12. Anderson S, Bloom KJ, Vallera DU, et al. Multisite analytic performance studies of a real-time polymerase chain reaction assay for the detection of BRAF V600E mutations in formalin-fixed, paraffin-embedded tissue specimens of malignant melanoma. Arch Pathol Lab Med. 2012;136(11):1385–91.
13. Curtin JA, Busam K, Pinkel D, Bastian BC. Somatic activation of KIT in distinct subtypes of melanoma. J Clin Oncol. 2006;24(26):4340–6.
14. Carvajal RD, Antonescu CR, Wolchok JD, et al. KIT as a therapeutic target in metastatic melanoma. JAMA. 2011;305(22):2327–34.
15. Kim KB, Alrwas A. Treatment of KIT-mutated metastatic mucosal melanoma. Chin Clin Oncol. 2014;3(3):35.
16. Glatz-Krieger K, Glatz D, Mihatsch MJ. Virtual slides: high-quality demand, physical limitations, and affordability. Hum Pathol. 2003;34:968–74.
17. Gimbel DC, et al. A static-image telepathology system for dermatopathology consultation in East Africa: the Massachusetts General Hospital Experience. J Am Acad Dermatol. 2012;67(5):997–1007.
18. Giambrone D, et al. Obstacles hindering the mainstream practice of teledermatopathology. J Am Acad Dermatol. 2014;71(4):772–80.
19. Massone C, Brunasso AM, Campbell TM, Soyer HP. State of the art of teledermatopathology. Am J Dermatopathol. 2008;30:446–50.
20. Abbas O, Bhawan J. Infections in Dermatopathology: emerging frontiers. Am J Dermatopathol. 2012;34:789–96.
21. Molina-Ruiz AM, Santonja C, Rütten A, et al. Immunohistochemistry in the diagnosis of cutaneous viral infections-part I. Cutaneous viral infections by herpesviruses and papillomaviruses. Am J Dermatopathol. 2015;37:1–14.
22. Nikkels AF, Piérard GE. Perineal herpes simplex infection in bedridden geriatric patients. Am J Clin Dermatol. 2007;8:79–83.
23. Nikkels AF, Debrus S, Sadzot-Delvaux C, et al. Comparative immunohistochemical study of herpes simplex and varicella-zoster infections. Virchows Arch A Pathol Anat Histopathol. 1993;422:121–6.
24. Nikkels AF, Debrus S, Sadzot-Delvaux C, et al. Immunohistochemical identification of varicella-zoster virus gene 63-encoded protein (IE63) and late (gE) protein on smears and cutaneous biopsies: implications for diagnostic use. J Med Virol. 1995;47:342–7.
25. Cheuk W, Wong KO, Wong CS, et al. Immunostaining for human herpesvirus 8 latent nuclear antigen-1 helps distinguish Kaposi sarcoma from its mimickers. Am J Clin Pathol. 2004;121:335–42.
26. Robin YM, Guillou L, Michels JJ, et al. Human herpesvirus 8 immunostaining: a sensitive and specific method for diagnosing Kaposi sarcoma in paraffin-embedded sections. Am J Clin Pathol. 2004;121:330–4.
27. Kumar A, Singh S, Salhan S, et al. Evaluation of a developed species-specific monoclonal antibody for detecting Chlamydia trachomatis infections in endocervical specimens from female patients. Hybridoma (Larchmt). 2007;26:333–7.
28. Phelps RG, Knispel J, Tu ES, et al. Immunoperoxidase technique for detecting spirochetes in tissue sections: comparison with other methods. Int J Dermatol. 2000;39:609–13.

Chapter 7
Genomics, Ethics, and Compliance

Sara W. Faulks and Steven R. Feldman

Abstract Genomics offers unprecedented opportunity to personalize medical care. Pharmacogenomics may help identify the best treatments for patients. These advances raise new ethical issues to consider. These issues also interface with the critically important issue of patient adherence and compliance to treatment. This chapter begins with a review of the history of ethics and especially its relationship to research in medicine, and this is followed by a discussion of genomics and the ethical issues it elucidates, as well as compliance in medicine and the associated ethical implications. The chapter is concluded with a commentary regarding this rather contemporary movement of pharmacogenomics, which embodies both ethics and compliance and is pertinent to the field of dermatology.

Keywords Adherence • Compliance • Pharmacogenomics • Ethics • Genomics

History of Ethics in Research

This first section is a brief look at the history underlying the ethics that guide research today. It is important to understand from where ethical principles were birthed and why these basic principles are crucial before one can fully apply them in research and practice (Table 7.1) [1–6].

The Nuremberg Code

Ubiquitously considered in the field of research medicine to be one of, if not the most significant document in the foundation of objective ethical principles, the Nuremberg Code is a landmark document that arose in 1947 from a dark history.

S.W. Faulks, BS • S.R. Feldman, MD, PhD (✉)
Department of Dermatology, Wake Forest Baptist Medical Center,
4618 Country Club Road, Winston-Salem, NC 27104, USA
e-mail: sfeldman@wakehealth.edu

R.A. Norman (ed.), *Personalized, Evolutionary, and Ecological Dermatology*,
DOI 10.1007/978-3-319-41088-3_7

Table 7.1 Historical documents and major contributions to ethics

Document	Major contributions
The Nuremberg Code, 1947	Cornerstone of objective ethical principles; establishes informed consent and the right to withdraw
Geneva Declaration, 1948	A revised and more contemporary Hippocratic Oath; a pledge that the physician's first priority is to give his or her life to serve humanity
Declaration of Helsinki, 1964	Ever-evolving document, loosens the previously very strict principles of informed consent and right to withdraw, differentiates between research with a direct therapeutic benefit versus an indirect and more generalized scientific benefit
Belmont Report, 1979	Details respect for persons, beneficence, and justice, and their respective associations with informed consent, assessment of risks and benefits, and selection of subjects
CIOMS, 1993	Particularly focuses on maintaining ethical standards in research in less developed countries and ensuring informed consent is adequately obtained given cultural differences

During World War Two, concentration camp prisoners were subjected to atrocities against their will, those atrocities including coercion by Nazi physicians – physicians who by the nature of their training were supposed to help patients and certainly do no harm – to participate in dangerous medical research [1]. The research was not benign, often leaving the prisoners severely deformed, and death was a common fate. Twenty German physicians in total, in addition to three adminstrators, were indicted in 1946 for these acts and tried by the International Military Tribunal, which was comprised of judges from the four allied powers (the United States, Britain, France, and the former Soviet Union), in what came to be known as the Doctors' Trial. The defense maintained that the physicians had not acted beyond the limits of any accepted standards for that time in terms of medical experiments on humans and went further to contend that the doctors were not brutal murderers but that their actions in fact were rather "a brutalizing effect of the war" [1].

What came of the trial was more than the final verdict and fate of these physicians. The judges saw an opportunity and need for reform in the regulation of the research of human subjects. They believed that the Hippocratic tradition – that of physician *self*-regulation of skills and ethics that were learned during proper medical training – was not enough to protect human subjects; what was needed was a defined set of medical principles not for the physicians but for the human subjects, to ensure their wellbeing, and this was the cornerstone of the development of the Nuremberg Code which "stipulates that no one may be part of a medical experiment without competent informed consent and the right to withdraw this consent at any point during the experiment" [1].

Although the Nuremberg Code has not been deemed law by any particular country, it nonetheless serves as the foundation of ethical principles that protect human research subjects in that it merges the principles of the Hippocratic ethics, which should in theory guide all physicians to do no harm, with the objective protection of human subjects through informed consent; not only does the Code ensure that the best interest of the subject is taken into account by the physician, but it also gives the subject the right to protect him or herself, and very importantly, it gives the human subject equal power in terminating his or her role in an experiment when it is no longer in that person's best interest [2].

The Geneva Declaration

Soon after the creation of the Nuremberg Code, the World Medical Association (WMA) met in 1948 with the purpose of creating a modernized alternative to the Hippocratic Oath, a document whose reputation for holding doctors to high ethical standards had begun to deteriorate after the gross misconduct of Nazi doctors in World War Two; the Geneva Declaration ensued. Considered a revised and more contemporary Hippocratic Oath, it is a pledge that the physician's first priority is to give his or her life to serve humanity [7]. Distinctively, the Geneva Declaration makes no specific reference to religion, abolishes antiquated references to, for example, "ancient slave doctors" or "lithocystotomies", and especially emphasizes the physician's duty to avoid influence by nationality, race, politics, or social status [8].

The Declaration of Helsinki

In 1964 the WMA adopted the Declaration of Helsinki, another landmark document in the evolution of medical ethics. Though the original Declaration of Helsinki hailed from the preceding Nuremberg Code, there were some notable distinctions: as opposed to an explicitly strict rule that only the research subject may give his or her own consent to participate in a study, the Declaration of Helsinki allowed for the subject's legal guardian to give consent if the subject was legally incapable (as in the case of a child or a comatose person, for example), and an ambiguous statement in the Nuremberg Code regarding the subject electing to withdraw from a study was clarified by adding that the investigator may also discontinue the study if the subject is not mentally capable to, unable to, or does not choose to withdraw consent [3]. The Declaration also differentiated between clinical research with a therapeutic benefit for patients versus clinical research that was solely scientific, without specific therapeutic patient benefit, and this distinction remained part of the Declaration until the Edinburgh revision in 2000 [3]. The Declaration, indeed, focuses on guidance of the physician involved in human research with specific focus on the responsibility to protect the human research subjects; but furthermore, its slight relaxation of the rules of informed consent, such as allowing parents to consent for their children in vaccine research, was an early nod toward public health and furthering scientific knowledge for the benefit of all of humanity [9].

The Declaration of Helsinki, a key historical element in defining the rights of human research subjects, even upon which the United States has based its regulations defining ethical conduct in research with human subjects, has become a sort of ever-changing and evolving document which has been revised several times from the original version to reflect the contemporary state of an always advancing field of medicine and medical research [10]. The beauty of the Declaration of Helsinki lies in that is was written by physicians as essential, nonnegotiable ethical standards to guide their practice as one of the early efforts to internationally regulate ethical standards with objective criteria in an accessible, relatively succinct composition of principles [11].

The Belmont Report

After the devastating Tuskegee Syphilis Study in the United States, the National Commission for the Protection of Human Subjects of Biomedical and Behavioral Research was formed to first determine and specify ethical principles and afterward to generate instructions that ensure and aid with adherence to these ethical principles; with these recommendations, the Belmont Report was published in the United States in 1979 [12]. The ethical principles in the Belmont Report are used to resolve potential ethical problems in the research of human subjects and include three key principles—respect for persons, beneficence, and justice— associated with informed consent, assessment of risks and benefits, and selection of subjects, respectively (Table 7.2) [4, 13].

Informed consent in the Belmont Report is more specifically defined as the research subject comprehending – though the determination of who is truly comprehending is not defined – the nature of the study, as well as its risks, benefits, and alternatives, and not being coerced into participation in a study beyond what would be considered reasonable influence [14]. Furthermore, regarding subjects who cannot give their own informed consent, such as children or comatose patients, the Belmont Report suggests that a third party be appointed to make the decision in the person's best interest [14]. Informed consent applies to the principle of respect for persons in which the research subject is autonomous and has the right to maintain his or her dignity, all attainable on the basis that a competent person is properly informed and elects participation of his or her own will [15].

Assessment of risks and benefits in the Belmont Report refers to the obligation to assess the likelihood of any risk and to estimate the severity of each risk, as well as the benefits, which can be more generalized, such as a benefit for humanity through the advancement of medicine [14]. Assessment of risks and benefits applies to the principle of beneficence as outlined in the Belmont Report, which specifies

Table 7.2 Ethical principles in the Belmont report and respective associations

Principle	Association
Respect for persons	Informed consent
Beneficence	Assessment of risks and benefits
Justice	Selection of subjects

doing what is good for the patient by ensuring that the risks of the research are minimal relative to the potential benefits [15].

Selection of subjects focuses on the fair selection of participants in terms of equal opportunity for all people to have access to the benefits and also, of course, the risks of research [14]. Selection of subjects applies to the principle of justice in the Belmont Report in that the people selected for research must have equal chance of bearing the brunt of the research's risks as well as gaining from its benefits, and research is totally inexcusable if it focuses on a specific group of people simply due to easier access of those participants [15].

Again, the Belmont Report was a response due to outrage and concern over the nature of research after the Tuskegee Syphilis Study, and the purpose of the Report was to organize ideas about the ethics of research on human subjects into discrete principles, as well as model the "moral demands" that stem from these ethical matters in research [16].

The International Ethical Guidelines for Biomedical Research Involving Human Subjects

In 1949 the Council for International Organizations of Medical Sciences was formed by the World Health Organization and the United Nations Educational, Scientific, and Cultural Organization (UNESCO) as a global, non-governmental institution to assist the biomedical sciences in international health policies and ethics [17]. A particular focus of the organization is on ethics related to biomedical research, and the organization has released several sets of guidelines, including the Proposed International Ethical Guidelines for Biomedical Research Involving Human Subjects in 1982, the International Guidelines for Ethical Review of Epidemiological Studies in 1991, and finally the International Ethical Guidelines for Biomedical Research Involving Human Subjects (better known as "CIOMS") in 1993, which has since been revised most recently in 2002 and includes a general remark about ethical guidelines as well as a preamble and 21 guidelines, all of which are especially relevant to poorer countries and focus on objectively specifying the ethics of biomedical research, implementing these ethics, and instituting methods to audit adherence to ethics in research involving human subjects [18]. The CIOMS is unique in its particular focus on maintaining ethical standards in research in less developed countries and ensuring informed consent is adequately obtained given cultural differences [5].

Genomics and Genetics

While genetics refers to the study of specific genes potentially involved in disease processes, genomics is a newer field, a much more encompassing term which refers to the study of the entire set of a human's genes – the genome – and its understandably extensive yet complicated involvement in disease processes.

The link between genomics and public health was highlighted in the 1990s with the Human Genome Project, and the international perspective is totally dependent on the partnership of multiple nations and multiple global organizations such as the World Health Organization and UNESCO working together toward a common goal of advancing medicine and hence advancing humanity; specifically, the public health goal as it relates to genomics is to, through the study of genetic and environmental factors including social and political factors leading to disease, craft successful strategies that focus on altering environmental factors with a goal of inhibiting or treating disease in people with specific genomic predispositions [19].

Ethical Issues Related to Genomics

As could be surmised, the ethical issues concerning genomics are copious and steadily unfolding as the field grows. The basic ethical principles, first modernly defined in the Nuremberg Code and further specified and matured for decades thereafter, serve as a source of reason in delineating these sometimes quite perplexing issues.

Informed Consent and the Right to Withdraw

The heart of ethics in the research of human subjects, as discussed at the beginning of the chapter, lies in obtaining informed consent from the subject to ensure that the participant entirely understands all risks and benefits of the research. However, in genomic research there are some inherent limits to obtaining informed consent. Especially since there is negligible significant immediate clinical consequence of a blood draw in gathering genomic information on an individual, the risks of genomic sequencing and research currently remain largely unknown; genomics is more of a collaborative result from gathering large amounts of genomic information on many individuals, so the question of re-consent is relative, as there is the real possibility of genomic data being used at a time in the future for research purposes that are different from the original intent of the data – and even further muddling this issue of informed consent is that a participant's genomic information can very well have implications for a family member with whom he or she most certainly shares significant biological information, and the family member likely would not have originally consented to be part of the research study [20]. To curb the confounding issue of informed consent, it is suggested to openly discuss with the participant while obtaining consent specifically what information he or she would like to have and to modify the research of that genomic information to be more or less limited, and it is recommended to discuss and determine any desired future interaction there should be between researcher and participant regarding significant genomic findings that could potentially be discovered in the future [21].

As the right of informed consent in genomic research is an essential concept, yet sometimes difficult to obtain, the right of research subjects to withdraw from genomic research too is an important and also quite problematic one. In biobanking, for example, if every participant could potentially decide to withdraw his or her sample from the data set, this would undermine the entire concept of biobanks, which hinge on gathering and maintaining huge collections of large amounts of samples; the sudden withdrawal of data would abate the power and significance of the biobank and, furthermore, would squander valuable resources [22]. Another problematic reason regarding withdrawal in biobanking is the simple impossibility of withdrawing a person's sample once the data has been published [23].

Confidentiality and Privacy

Though confidentiality and privacy are traditionally ensured in research through the use of de-identification of data, securing of personal information, regulation of access, and placement of firewalls, these methods have attracted growing concern regarding the adequate protection of privacy in genomic research [24]. The fact that information will remain confidential is stated during the process of informed consent, but in genomic research this concept is not always so simple. A subject's genetic information could reveal information that the person may prefer remain private from family members, employers, and insurance companies, including potential devastating disease processes or even misattributed paternity in some cases; though the information is often not clinically implicating, advancing technologies have nonetheless allowed for tiny amounts of genetic information from a subject to be able to identify that individual, or in the least reveal enough information so as that person's identification can be assumed, and this new possibility raises the important concern of the feasibility of maintaining patient privacy in genomic research [25].

For now, it is recommended to be as unequivocally clear as possible with research participants in terms of who will have the right to access their data and for what purposes it will be used, especially in an effort to maintain a circle of trust with the research subjects, who could very well already be wary of such research participation due to historical events such as those mentioned at the beginning of the chapter [26].

Return of Results

There is significant discrepancy in feedback that research participants receive based on their genomic findings, as there is little consensus regarding not only if data will be returned to the subject, but what data will be returned, and especially if there is an exception that incidentally found medically harmful findings should *always* be returned; there is currently no general agreement, and determining if one should, and if so how to, return these findings to the participants depends on several factors, including the intent of the particular study in which the subject is involved, standardized views about the subject's autonomy in deciding whether or not he or she prefers to know the results, and empirical data about the participants' psychological impacts as well as impacts on their medical care [27]. Although there is general accordance that a participant's consent should include dialogue about the real possibility of incidental findings in that person's genome, controversy still remains regarding which pieces of data that are incidentally found should be disclosed and if there are any which should always be disclosed to the subject [28]. Since genomics is a constantly evolving field, and there is currently such diversity in the way that results, especially incidental ones, are returned to participants, it is crucial that standardized views and practices are established to serve as guidance on feedback to participants about information that is potentially vital to their health [27].

Several suggestions have been proposed to alleviate the concerning issues of returning results to research subjects. Qualified disclosure, which is returning information to the subject that could be medically treated or prevented, as well as ensuring prudency when disclosing incidental information about minors, and preemptively limiting the incidental findings before the research so as to avoid ever finding them are all ways to help mitigate the issue [29]. An "automatized filtering system" is a potential real solution – though also somewhat ethically controversial as it promotes beneficence but somewhat undermines patient autonomy – to the dilemma, as it would allow for others to make decisions to return data without either the participant or the researcher being informed of every single decision, which in turn saves time of the researcher or physician, saves money, and limits potentially confusing information to a patient to only that information that is deemed significant [29]. A system is necessary to balance the research participant's right to have access to his or her own genetic data, the researcher's duties of nonmaleficence and beneficence, and hindrances related to time and money [30].

Therapeutic Misconception Regarding Benefits

The purpose of genomic research is somewhat unique. It is delineated in the process of informed consent and focuses on advancing medicine for the benefit of humanity via gathering and analyzing data, as opposed to directly benefitting the particular research subject involved; a well-documented misunderstanding of this matter lies in a fallacy known as "therapeutic misconception", where the research subject incorrectly expects his or her participation in the research to have a direct and personal therapeutic benefit, as opposed to a more generalized and indirect benefit to the public by advancing science [31]. Subjects can be confused about the goal of the research, how individualized it will be, and what direct benefits they will receive, and scales for therapeutic misconception have been suggested to recognize the subjects with inclinations for these misunderstandings so as to preemptively rectify their misinterpretations, as well as to encourage research regarding these therapeutic misconceptions and how to best curtail them through less ambiguous informed consent processes [32].

Patient Compliance

Patient compliance is the ability of a patient to follow his or her prescribed medical regimen, especially prescribed medications; noncompliance reduces the clinical utility of a potentially highly efficacious drug if a patient does not take it (and can result in side effects if used in greater than recommended amounts), and this can result in severe medical consequences for the patient, a wasting of financial resources, as well as inaccurate data in clinical trials [33]. Patient noncompliance can be a primary explanation for treatment failure in patients. The term "adherence" is accepted and used by some as a less judgmental alternative to the words "compliance" or "concordance", as this term avoids focus on blame or accusation of the patient [34].

Barriers to Compliance

Barriers to patient compliance are numerous (see below). These barriers include patients forgetting or misunderstanding the physician's recommendations, especially when given considerable volumes of information or when the patient's mood is anxious or displeased due to the care he or she received at the office visit; a lack of successful communication or trust in the patient-physician relationship; discordance between physician and patient where they lack a mutual understanding for each other and the patient is dissatisfied with involvement in his or her care; disparate views and attitudes between doctor and patient regarding illness and treatment as a consequence of cultural norms; and depression. These and many other factors can contribute to poor compliance: [35]

- Forgetting recommendations
- Misunderstanding recommendations
- Lack of trust in patient-physician relationship
- Lack of mutual understanding between patient and physician
- Patient dissatisfaction with care
- Disparate views and attitudes due to cultural norms
- Patient depression

Interventions to Improve Compliance

Many interventions have been suggested to improve compliance (see below), and research regarding this topic is ongoing, as there is no convincing evidence of any one particular intervention's superiority. Monetary reward has been suggested as a potential means of curtailing patient noncompliance, and some very preliminary data suggests that it modestly does improve patient compliance, though it is important, of course, to note that the monetary reward for the patient need not outprice the monetary gain associated with better compliance; for example, monetary rewards for tuberculosis treatment compliance would result in net positive monetary gain ultimately, hence benefitting both the patient's health and the general public's resources [36].

Unfortunately, studies examining interventions such as increasing daily support from family members, peers, and medical professionals and directed education and counseling have generally resulted in insufficient evidence regarding these specific interventions to improve compliance; the studies also fail to conclude accurate methods to assess compliance and, even so, are largely characterized by inadequate population sizes to be able to deduce significant results [37]. The more present-day act of patients' use of Internet research affecting their compliance has been questioned as a factor altering their adherence, but newer research into this question actually indicates that a much more convincing factor than the Internet is simply the quality of the physician in terms of competence, compassion, and communication skills [38].

Although research regarding the optimum tactics to ensure patient compliance have historically revealed scant data, there are nonetheless several related considerations that have been exposed and deemed influential, which include accurate appraisal of the patient's comprehension of the medical regimen, explicit and unambiguous communication between doctor and patient, and support of and confidence in the relationship between the physician and patient [35]. Communication between doctor and patient is a factor that has a particularly positive impact on patient compliance, so it is wise for physicians to strive to improve their abilities to communicate with all patients from different backgrounds, views, and cultures in order to ameliorate patient compliance [39]. Communication strategies wholly inclusive of cognitive, behavioral, and emotional tactics have shown relative superior effectiveness when compared with unidirectional approaches [40].

Interventions studied to improve compliance:

- Communication strategies wholly inclusive of cognitive, behavioral, and emotional tactics [40]
- Daily peer support [37]
- Education [37]
- Counseling [37]
- Monetary reward [36]

Compliance, Ethics, and Pharmacogenomics: Putting It All Together

Pharmacogenomics is relatively new, as technological advances have made it possible, through genomic research, to discover how drugs will affect certain patients based on their particular genomes. By being able to identify what drugs will best treat a patient, treatments may be more effective, may reduce the time patients suffer, and may help control costs otherwise wasted on ineffective measures. Pharmacogenomics raises issues of ethics as well as compliance. Many medical fields, including dermatology, are expanding targeted treatment options for patients by using pharmacogenomic technologies, which are now available. This final section of the chapter will acknowledge several examples of pharmacogenomic research advancing dermatology and will conclude with a consideration of the connection with ethics and compliance.

Severe cutaneous adverse reactions to medications – such as Stevens-Johnson syndrome, toxic epidermal necrolysis, and drug reaction with associated eosinophilia and systemic symptoms (DRESS) – are relatively rare but potentially fatal. Immune and non-immune gene pathways may be involved. Pharmacogenomic markers have been discovered that identify patients with genetic predispositions to not clear or not metabolize a drug adequately, with particular HLA-associated hypersensitivities to certain drugs, and with certain protein-protein binding tendencies. The markers can help patients avoid those offending agents, which could have devastatingly harmful adverse effects on them [41].

Phenytoin is an antiepileptic drug that has a potential adverse effect of cutaneous reactions, ranging from mild drug rash to potentially life-threatening Stevens-Johnson syndrome, toxic epidermal necrolysis, and DRESS [42]. CYP2C variants have been identified, especially CYP2C9*3, which are associated with a reduced clearance of phenytoin and an increased susceptibility to adverse reactions, especially these adverse cutaneous manifestations. These discoveries have stimulated the launch of further research into more practical tests to identify these patients prior to their initiation of treatment with phenytoin [42].

Pharmacoepigenetics has gained a presence in the study of treatments for systemic lupus erythematosus (SLE) and is responsible for the development of innovative, new therapies such as anti-miRNA drugs and histone modification histone deacetylase (HDAC) inhibitors; the advances that new genomic technology has contributed to the study of pharmacogenomics in SLE are pivotal, since this disease is such a diverse one and therefore will require ongoing genomic research to pinpoint unknown markers for susceptibility to the disease, for diagnosis of the disease, and especially for pharmacologic treatment of the disease in terms of the best efficacy and fewest adverse effects [43].

Pharmacogenomics is even playing a role in aesthetic dermatology, both in determining the intrinsic properties of young skin that make it appear youthful and hence can facilitate the development of age-defying cosmetics, as well as in determining the ingredients most effective in counteracting photoaging; and beyond *pharmaco*genomics, genomics continues to play a part in studying dermatologic cancers and identifying the natural skin protective qualities that are inherent in some individuals yet appear deficient in others with similar skin types and sun-exposure history [44].

This chapter has alluded to the relationship of ethics and compliance with pharmacogenomics, but it is nevertheless important to explicitly specify these connections (Fig. 7.1). The study of pharmacogenomics relies upon a multitude of research

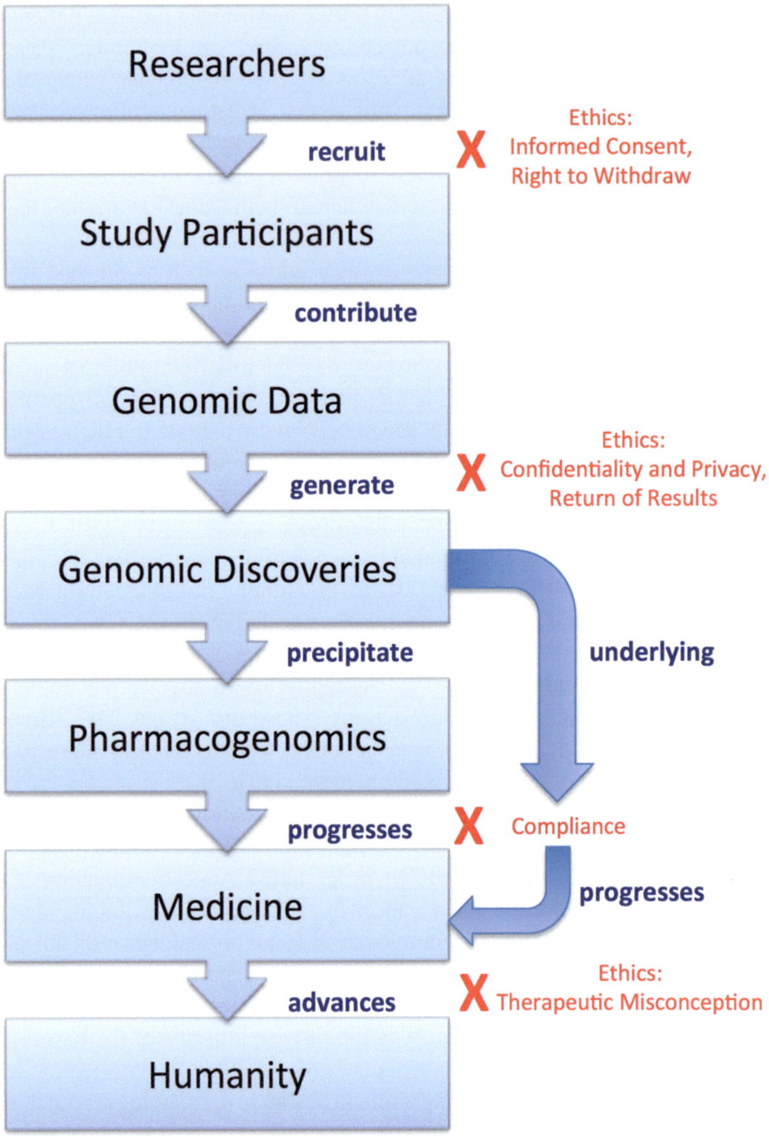

Fig. 7.1 Relationships between ethics, genetics and compliance. Researchers recruit study participants who contribute their genomic data, which in turn generates genomic discoveries which have precipitated the field of pharmacogenomics. This progresses medicine and, ultimately, advances humanity. Ethical issues such as informed consent and the right to withdraw can mar the recruitment process; confidentiality and privacy and return of results can complicate the generation of genomic discoveries; and therapeutic misconception can confuse participants' ideas regarding the advancement of all of humanity. Poor compliance, too, can impede the pharmacogenomics research and the translation of that research into clinical practice. Genomic discoveries that underlie and, therefore, determine compliance may one day lead to new understandings of patient behavior and better ways to improve patients' treatment outcomes

subjects to contribute their genomic information to allow for progress in identifying genomic predispositions to drugs and adverse effects of drugs. Certainly, participation in this type of research can elicit any and all of the ethical issues related to genomic research that are detailed in the chapter. Compliance plays another role in that if the subject is noncompliant in pharmacogenomic studies, this can totally undermine the entire outcome of the investigation. An intriguing thought is the possibility of one day learning the genetic factors that determine compliance. A common question is, "Is it ethical to expect compliance and life-style changes without considering the impact on a person's life?" [45]. The answer is that one *must* consider the impact on a person's life. Recognize the impact, mitigate the impact, and follow up on the impact. Foster a relationship with the patient. This is the ethical solution that encourages compliance – and *that* is the goal.

References

1. Freyhofer HH. The Nuremberg Medical Trial. New York: Peter Lang Publishing; 2004. p. 10–11.
2. Gillon R. Medical oaths, declarations, and codes. Br Med J (Clin Res Ed). 1985; 290(6476):1194–5.
3. Carlson R, Boyd KM, Webb DJ. The revision of the Declaration of Helsinki: past, present and future. Br J Clin Pharmacol. 2004;57(6):695–713.
4. U.S. Department of Health and Human Services. The Belmont report. http://www.hhs.gov/ohrp/humansubjects/guidance/belmont.html. Accessed 2015 June.
5. Brody BA. The Ethics of Biomedical Research: An International Perspective. New York: Oxford University Press; 1998. p. 36.
6. Shuster E. Fifty years later: the significance of the Nuremberg code. N Engl J Med. 1997;337:1436–40.
7. Gillon R. Medical oaths, declarations, and codes. Br Med J (Clin Res Ed). 1985; 290(6476):1194–5.
8. Frewer A. Human rights from the Nuremberg doctors trial to the Geneva declaration. Persons and institutions in medical ethics and history. Med Health Care Philos. 2010;13(3):259–68.
9. Williams JR. The Declaration of Helsinki and public health. Bulletin of the World Health Organization. 2008;86(8):650–2.
10. Holt GR. Declaration of Helsinki-the world's document of conscience and responsibility. South Med J. 2014;107(7):407.
11. Parsa-Parsi RW, Ellis R, Wiesing U. Fifty years at the forefront of ethical guidance: the world medical association declaration of Helsinki. South Med J. 2014;107(7):405–6.
12. Mandal J, Acharya S, Parija SC. Ethics in human research. Trop Parasitol. 2011;1(1):2–3.
13. Breault JL. Protecting human research subjects: the past defines the future. Ochsner J. 2006;6(1):15–20.
14. Fischer BA. A summary of important documents in the field of research ethics. Schizophr Bull. 2006;32(1):69–80.
15. Beauchamp TL. The Belmont report. The Oxford textbook of clinical research ethics. New York: Oxford University Press; 2011. p. 149–155.
16. Vollmer SH, Howard G. Statistical power, the Belmont report, and the ethics of clinical trials. Sci Eng Ethics. 2010;16(4):675–91.
17. About us. Council for International Organizations of Medical Sciences. http://www.cioms.ch/index.php/2012-06-07-19-16-08/about-us. Accessed 2015 June.
18. International Ethical Guidelines for Biomedical Research Involving Human Subjects. Geneva. 2002. http://www.cioms.ch/publications/layout_guide2002.pdf. Accessed 2015 June.

19. Stewart A, Karmali M, Zimmern R. GRaPH Int: a International Network for Public Health Genomics. In: Knoppers BA, editor. Genomics and public health: legal and socio-ethical perspectives. Leiden: Martinus Nijhoff; 2006. p. 260.
20. Caulfield T, McGuire AL, Cho M, Buchanan JA, Burgess MM, Danilczyk U, et al. Research ethics recommendations for whole-genome research: consensus statement. PLoS Biol. 2008;6(3):e73.
21. Ayuso C, Millan JM, Mancheno M, Dal-Re R. Informed consent for whole-genome sequencing studies in the clinical setting. Proposed recommendations on essential content and process. Eur J Hum Genet. 2013;21(10):1054–9.
22. Holm S. Withdrawing from research: a rethink in the context of research biobanks. Health Care Anal. 2011;19(3):269–81.
23. Boddington P. Ethical challenges in genomics research: a guide to understanding ethics in context. New York: Springer; 2012. p. 91.
24. Kaye J. The tension between data sharing and the protection of privacy in genomics research. Annu Rev Genomics Hum Genet. 2012;13:415–31.
25. Kaye J, Boddington P, de Vries J, Hawkins N, Melham K. Ethical implications of the use of whole genome methods in medical research. Eur J Hum Genet. 2010;18(4):398–403.
26. Lin Z, Owen AB, Altman RB. Genetics. Genomic research and human subject privacy. Science. 2004;305(5681):183.
27. Henderson GE, Wolf SM, Kuczynski KJ, Joffe S, Sharp RR, Parsons DW, et al. The challenge of informed consent and return of results in translational genomics: empirical analysis and recommendations. J Law Med Ethics. 2014;42(3):344–55.
28. Clarke AJ. Managing the ethical challenges of next-generation sequencing in genomic medicine. Br Med Bull. 2014;111(1):17–30.
29. Christenhusz GM, Devriendt K, Dierickx K. To tell or not to tell? A systematic review of ethical reflections on incidental findings arising in genetics contexts. Eur J Hum Genet. 2013;21(3):248–55.
30. Klitzman R, Appelbaum PS, Fyer A, Martinez J, Buquez B, Wynn J, et al. Researchers' views on return of incidental genomic research results: qualitative and quantitative findings. Genet Med. 2013;15(11):888–95.
31. Pinxten W, Howard HC. Ethical issues raised by whole genome sequencing. Best Pract Res Clin Gastroenterol. 2014;28(2):269–79.
32. Appelbaum PS, Anatchkova M, Albert K, Dunn LB, Lidz CW. Therapeutic misconception in research subjects: development and validation of a measure. Clin Trials. 2012;9(6):748–61.
33. Kermani F, Davies M. Patient compliance: sweetening the pill. Hampshire: Gower; 2006.
34. McDonald HP, Garg AX, Haynes RB. Interventions to enhance patient adherence to medication prescriptions. J Am Med Assoc. 2002;288(22):2868–79.
35. Martin LR, Williams SL, Haskard KB, DiMatteo MR. The challenge of patient adherence. Ther Clin Risk Manag. 2005;1(3):189–99.
36. Giuffrida A, Torgerson DJ. Should we pay the patient? Review of financial incentives to enhance patient compliance. BMJ. 1997;315(7110):703–7.
37. Nieuwlaat R, Wilczynski N, Navarro T, Hobson N, Jeffery R, Keepanasseril A, et al. Interventions for enhancing medication adherence. Cochrane Database Syst Rev 2014;(11):CD000011.
38. Laugesen J, Hassanein K, Yuan Y. The impact of internet health information on patient compliance: a research model and empirical study. J Med Internet Res. 2015;17(6):e143.
39. Zolnierek KBH, DiMatteo MR. Physician communication and patient adherence to treatment: a meta-analysis. Med Care. 2009;47(8):826–34.
40. Roter DL, Hall JA, Merisca R, Nordstrom B, Cretin D, Svarstad B. Effectiveness of interventions to improve patient compliance: a meta-analysis. Med Care. 1998;36(8):1138–61.
41. Dao R, Su S, Chung W. Recent advances of pharmacogenomics in severe cutaneous adverse reactions: immune and nonimmune mechanisms. Asia Pac Allergy. 2015;5(2):59–67. doi:10.5415/apallergy.2015.5.2.59.

42. Chung W, Chang W, Lee Y, Wu Y, Yang C, Ho H, et al. Genetic variants associated with phenytoin-related severe cutaneous adverse reactions. J Am Med Assoc. 2014;312(5):525–34. doi:10.1001/jama.2014.7859.
43. Guo Y, Sawalha AH, Lu Q. Epigenetics in the treatment of systemic lupus erythematosus: potential clinical application. Clin Immunol. 2014;155(1):79–90. doi:10.1016/j.clim.2014.09.002.
44. Draelos ZD. Genomics: the future of cosmetic dermatology. J Cosmet Dermatol. 2010;9:265–6.
45. Bernardini J. Ethical issues of compliance/adherence in the treatment of hypertension. Adv Chronic Kidney Dis. 2004;11(2):222–7.

Chapter 8
Genetics, Nutrition, and Skin

Robert A. Norman, Asmi H. Sanghvi, and John Barksdale

Abstract Personalized nutrition is not a novel concept but the incorporation of nutrigenetics and nutrigenomics offers this field exciting new angles that could yield significant contributions to individual health. Nutrigenetics explores the way an individual's unique genome will respond to dietary nutrients while nutrigenomics explores the way dietary nutrients influences a person's genome. This chapter highlights the relevance to dermatology and specific dermatological conditions, concluding with a commentary on future considerations regarding nutrition, genetics, and skin.

Keywords Personalized nutrition • Dermatonutrigenomics • Dermagenetics • Nutrigenetics • Nutrigenomics

Personalized Nutrition and Dermatogenetics

Skin is the largest organ system of the human body. Skin type, hair color and other attributes are principally determined by genetic contributions from the parents to the fetus at conception. Additionally, prenatal nutrition and prenatal care of the expectant mother are important in all aspects of optimal intra-uterine fetal organ growth and development, including skin.

Genetics is defined by the World Health Organization as "the study of heredity" and genomics is defined "as the study of genes and their functions" [1, 2].

R.A. Norman, DO, MPH, MBA (✉)
Professor, Department of Dermatology, Nova Southeastern Medical School, Ft. Lauderdale, FL, USA

Dermatology Healthcare, 8002 Gunn Highway, Tampa, FL 33626, USA
e-mail: skindrrob@aol.com

A.H. Sanghvi, BS
OMS IV, Tampa, FL, USA

J. Barksdale
LMU-DCOM, OMS1, Nebraska, NE, USA

R.A. Norman (ed.), *Personalized, Evolutionary, and Ecological Dermatology*, DOI 10.1007/978-3-319-41088-3_8

Additionally, the World Health Organization states, "The main difference between genomics and genetics is that genetics scrutinizes the functioning and composition of the single gene whereas genomics addresses all genes and their inter-relationships in order to identify their combined influence on the growth and development of the organism" [1, 2].

Dermagenetics is the study of heredity pertaining specifically to skin, its derivatives (hair, nails) and appendages. As Subbiah points out, "The common mutations examined are related to the enzymes involved in the following: (a) collagen breakdown, (b) photoaging and free oxygen radical elimination, (c) degradation of environmental pollutants, and d) generation of pro-inflammatory molecules" [3, 4]. As defined by this author, (RAN), dermatonutrigenomics is the study of genes and nutrition and their interrelationships in order to identify their combined influence on the growth and development of the skin.

Nutrition, as defined by the World Health Organization, "is the intake of food, considered in relation to the body's dietary needs. Good nutrition – an adequate, well balanced diet combined with regular physical activity – is a cornerstone of good health. Poor nutrition and malnutrition can lead to reduced immunity, increased susceptibility to disease, impaired physical and mental development, and reduced productivity" [1, 2].

Personalized nutrition and disease prevention is not a novel concept. An association between diet and disease has persisted since the early days of the history of medicine. Natural products have been utilized for preventing several diseases including various forms of cancer. Hippocrates, the father of modern medicine, proclaimed "Let food be thy medicine and medicine be thy food." For decades nutritionists have been adjusting diets for their clients according to cultural needs, personal beliefs, and personal preferences. For example, there are those who desire a vegan diet and need education on the necessity of supplementing vitamins D and B12 to avoid any possible neurological deficits [4]. Likewise, medical physicians have long discovered certain stages of life and conditions that require a fine tuning of nutritional adjustments. These include the increased needs of a developing fetal brain, pregnant or lactating mother, or geriatric patient.

Nutrigenetics and nutrigenomics offer a further focused inspection of a person, down to the biochemical level of their genes, and allow a more intimate analysis of their nutrient requirements for optimal health. When a person's genetics are considered, both in how they react to nutrients and how nutrients react to their genomes, one may ultimately reach a position where chronic conditions, predisposed diseases, and what were once "inevitable" pathologies influenced by nutrition can potentially be stalled or even eradicated. This is truly an exciting endeavor for health care. While this emerging field has applications in all areas of medicine and healthcare, the topic under review is dermatology. Historically there has been an association between nutrition and skin allure, maturity, integrity, and health per biologic and biochemical processes [5]. Accordingly, the study of skin disease and personalized nutrition are inexplicably linked and will be explored in this chapter.

Nutrigenetics

Nutrigenetics is the study of how the genetic makeup of an individual determines their response to nutritional interventions [6]. This field observes whether a genome reacts or does not to various foods and dietary factors through analysis of polymorphisms and other genetic variations. These findings are then correlated with various disease states. Every genetic makeup is unique in some form, which causes some individuals to respond positively to some therapies whereas another individual may respond poorly, simply based on subtle difference in the amount or the type of DNA combinations. This is important to consider because some people have unique genes or mutations that predispose them to certain diseases, conditions, or susceptibilities.

Classifications

What makes one individual genetic make-up different from one another? The most common variation is found through SNPs, that is, single nucleotide polymorphisms. These SNPs account for 90 % of the genetic variation found from one individual to the next [7]. A SNP is a single DNA nucleotide, so SNP variations means that while in one individual there may be a stretch of DNA that codes for cytosine-thymine-alanine, another may have a single change in that DNA sequence such that the stretch codes for cytosine-cytosine-alanine. There are around 10 million SNPs in the human genome, and if the SNP occurs within a gene or even a regulatory region corresponding to a gene these may have an impact on proteins manifested by the genetic code, including whether that protein is expressed or not, how many copies are made, and what the structure of the protein is [7]. Research in the field of genetics has confirmed that SNPs are predictive of how an individual will respond to the environment, including drug reactions, toxin impact, and disease susceptibility.

The impact of SNPs can be direct or indirect. One study investigating the field of nutrigenetics found the influence of polymorphisms in the pathogenesis of occlusive heart disease, birth defects, and dementia [7]. It is known that nutritional deficiencies can disturb the normal regulation of one-carbon metabolism and homocystine hemostasis. This deficiency must be chronic and includes decreased availability of any of: folate, choline, methionine, vitamin B6, or vitamin B12. What the new research discovered was that certain individuals have a genetic polymorphism that actually works in a synergistic fashion with the above nutritional deficiencies that accelerates the disturbance of one-carbon metabolism and homocystine hemostasis to the point of leading to susceptibility to those medical conditions when the person is exposed to such a nutritional deficiency [8].

Applications

There are numerous dermatological conditions that are determined genetically- that is, they are inherited from parents and various combinations of alleles. A handful of these conditions can be abrogated through nutritional intervention. This is a good reason why nutrigenetics is so relevant to the field of dermatology. A few examples follow, with Table 8.1 describing the genetics and nutritional relevance.

Allergies

Allergies are extremely common, and general population studies have found that 25–30 % of households claim to have at least one family member who has a food allergy [9]. Food allergies are immunologic responses to foods, and the symptoms include anaphylaxis, dyspnea, and vomiting. Dermatologic findings include flushing, urticaria, angioedema, and ocular injection (see Figs. 8.1 and 8.2) [10]. A triad that runs in certain families includes atopic dermatitis, allergies, and asthma, reflecting a well-known finding that there is a genetic component to food allergies. Specifically, one study found that there is a 14-fold increase in the chance of having a peanut allergy if one has a family member with one [11]. Environmental factors also contribute to allergies, and therefore there may actually be a mix of genetic and environmental factors that manifest in food allergies. The best management for food allergies is a nutritionally focused one, that is, cessation of allergy-specific food consumption.

Table 8.1 Nutrition-genetics-skin

Disease	Skin	Genetics	Nutritional intervention
Food allergies	Urticaria	7 % increased chance of peanut allergy	Allergy specific elimination
Celiac disease	Dermatitis herpetiformis	HLA II genes	Gluten-free diet
Hartnup disease	Pellagra	Autosomal recessive	High protein diet
Phenylketonuria	Multiple (see text)	Autosomal recessive	Phenylalanine and aspartame-restricted diet

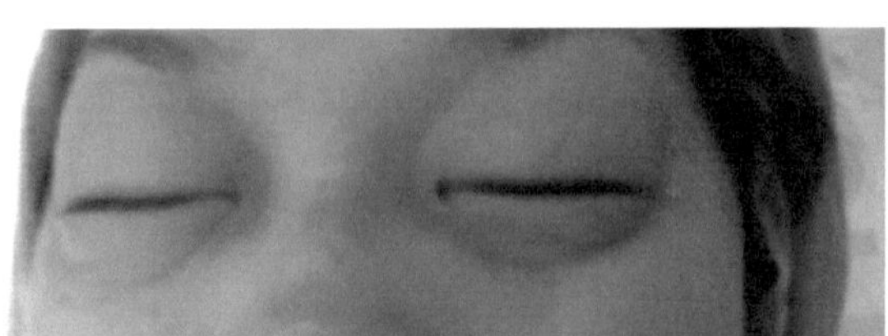

Fig. 8.1 Angioedema: food allergy reaction

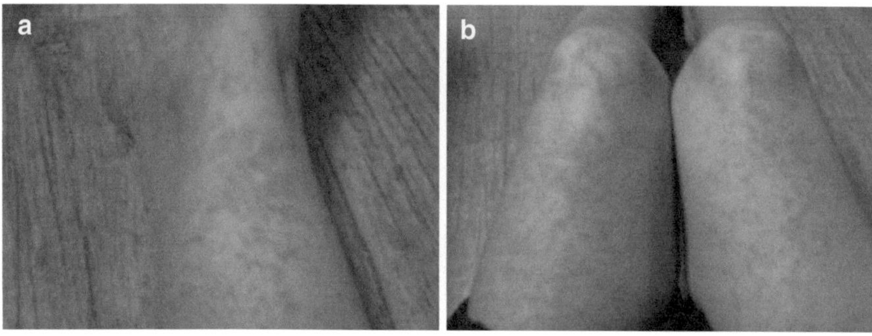

Fig. 8.2 (a, b) Urticaria: food allergy reaction

Celiac Disease

Celiac disease is a condition that has genetic, nutritional, and dermatological factors. It is an immune-mediated condition that predisposes an individual to have an adverse reaction to gluten products, which include wheat, rye, and barley [12]. The genetic component of celiac disease relates to specific HLA class II genes on chromosome 6, specifically variations of HLA-DQ2 and HLA-DQ8 [12]. Once again, just as with allergies, one is susceptible but not destined to develop celiac disease when they have these specific genetic variations. In fact, there is only 36–53 % increased risk associated with having either of these two genes, and there is an influential environmental contribution. The dermatological manifestations show up as dermatitis herpetiformis, an autoimmune blistering condition that improves with nutritional interventions that eliminate gluten from diet (Fig. 8.3) [13].

Inborn Errors of Metabolism

There are various metabolic conditions that also tie into the nutrition-genetics- dermatology connection. For example, Hartnup Disease is an autosomal recessive disorder in which the transportation of neutral amino acids across the intestinal border and kidney is grossly impaired (Fig. 8.4) [14]. The clinical manifestations of this hereditary disease include skin eruptions that resemble pellagra, cerebellar atacia, and aminoaciduria. Here, knowledge of biochemistry drives the nutritional-based treatment; a high protein diet is given to the patient, which serves to overcome the impairment [15]. Another well-known metabolic disorder is Phenylketonuria, which involves an autosomal recessive inheritance pattern and a defect in the metabolism of phenylalanine [16]. Aside from the common manifestations that include epilepsy, mental retardation, and the characteristic "musty" odor, there are several dermatological findings [17]. These include fair skin and hair, eczema, photosensitivity, increased pyogenic infections, increased keratosis pilaris, decreased pigmented nevi, alopecia, and scleroderma-like plaques. Intervention and treatment involve a phenylalanine and aspartame-restricted diet (Fig. 8.5) [18].

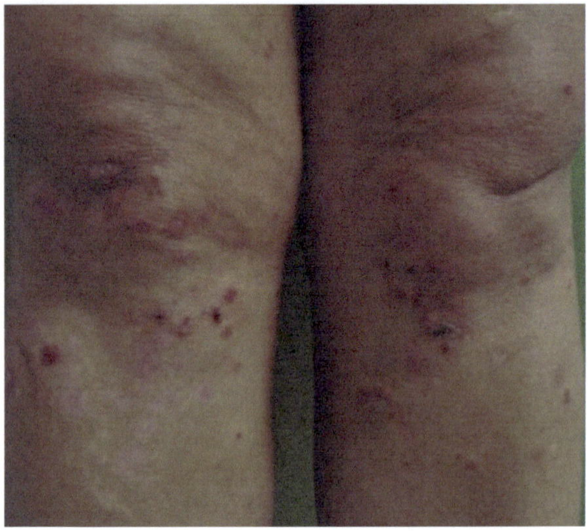

Fig. 8.3 Dermatitis herpetiformia: manifestation of celiac cisease

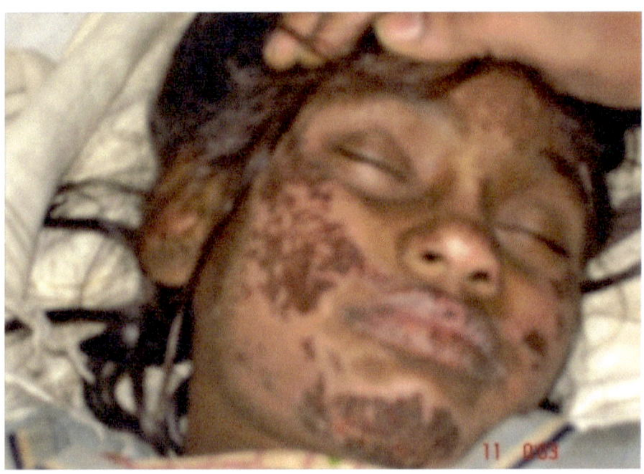

Fig. 8.4 Pellagra-like skin eruption: manifestation of Hartnup disease

Actinic Keratoses and Skin Cancers

A study performed by Halder et al demonstrated that tea polyphenols caused apoptosis in skin cancer cells and increased the activity of tumor suppression genes, which are key factors in the development of cutaneous melanoma [19]. In addition, they illuminated a probable mechanism for apoptosis induction and showed that the polyphenols did not cause an unfavorable outcome on the normal skin cells. This is a remarkable finding because it indicates that there may be a relatively low risk of adverse side effects from the use of polyphenols in primary cutaneous

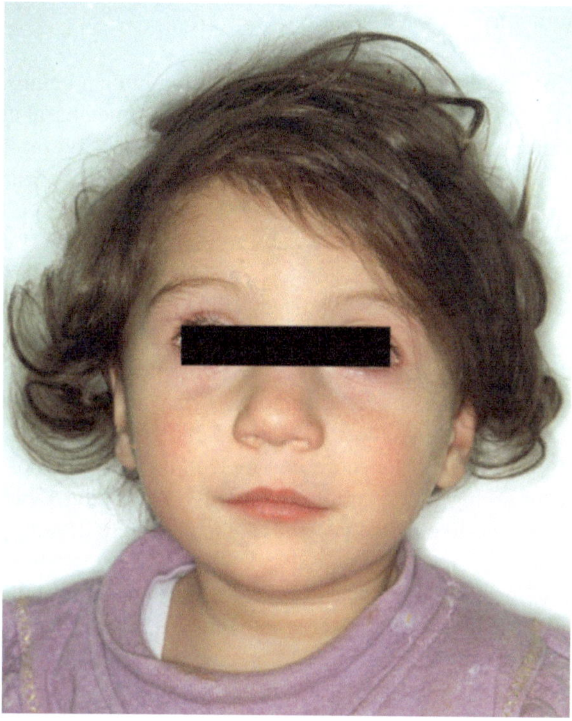

Fig. 8.5 Albino child with phenylketonuria

melanoma. Other researchers have shown a decrease in skin cancers based on green tea intake [20].

Actinic Keratosis

Actinic keratosis is a very common pre-malignant skin lesion consisting of a proliferation of abnormal ("dysplastic") cutaneous squamous cells (keratinocytes) in skin damaged by actinic (sun) radiation. Genetic factors also contribute to the development of actinic keratosis in that polymorphism in the p53 gene (located on chromosome 17) has been associated with increased incidence of actinic keratosis in families.

While avoidance of the damaging effects of the sun is the best way to prevent actinic keratoses, a low fat diet (21 % of dietary caloric intake) has also been shown to decrease the cumulative number of new actinic keratoses. In the study by Black et al [21], the cumulative number of new actinic keratoses per patient from months 4 through 24 was 10±13 in the control group and 3=/– in the low fat dietary intervention group.

Basal Cell Carcinoma

Basal cell carcinomas are the most common cancer in human beings. It is a malignant non-melanoma skin carcinoma arising from transformed basal cells of the epidermis. These tumors, if left untreated, may become locally aggressive and invade surrounding tissues and organs, especially in the head and neck where the tumors occur most frequently. Complete removal of a basal cell carcinoma is the goal of the many available modalities to treat basal cell carcinoma.

As with the prevention of actinic keratoses and squamous cell carcinomas of the skin, avoidance of new actinic (sun) damage is the primary line of prevention to the development of new basal cell carcinomas of the skin. Recently, vitamin B3 supplementation has been shown to also play a role in the prevention of non-melanoma (basal cell carcinoma, squamous cell carcinoma) skin cancers. Results gleaned from the Australian Oral Nicotinamide to Reduce Actinic Cancer (ONTRAC) Study showed patients who had two or more non-melanoma skin carcinomas during the preceding 5 years taking nicotinamide (Vitamin B3: 500 mg twice daily for 12 months) were 25 % less likely than peers taking a placebo to develop new basal cell carcinomas [22].

Environmental factors other than sun exposure may also contribute to the formation of BCC and SCC. Petroleum byproducts (e.g., asphalt, tar, soot, paraffin, and pitch), organophosphate compounds, and arsenic are all occupational exposures associated with cutaneous non-melanoma cancers [23–25].

Evidence exists that malfunctioning of the hedgehog (HH) signaling pathway and gene mutations increase the risk BCC development. The HH pathway influences differentiation of various tissues during fetal development. In adults, it continues to function in regulation of cell growth and differentiation. Malfunctioning of this pathway is associated with human malignancy, including BCC. The hedgehog gene in the HH pathway, codes for an extracellular protein, the sonic hedgehog (SHH) protein that binds to the cell membrane receptor complex to start a cascade of cellular events leading to cell proliferation [26].

The cell membrane receptor complex consists of two proteins: patched (PTCH)1 protein that is the ligand-binding component of the hedgehog receptor complex in the cell membrane smoothened (SMO) protein, that is responsible for transducing hedgehog signaling to downstream genes. In the resting state, PTCH1 holds SMO in an inactive state, thus inhibiting signaling to downstream genes. In the active state: SHH binds to PTCH1, PTCH1 inhibition of SMO is released and the hedgehog pathway is activated through a series of interacting proteins including suppressor of fused (SUFU) protein, leading in turn to the activation of transcription factors and to the expression of target cell cycle regulator genes [27].

A malfunctioning of the HH pathway is associated with human malignancy, including BCC. The normal functioning of the HH pathway can be disrupted because of mutations (changes in the genomic sequence i.e. the DNA sequence of the cell's genome) in the genes coding for the PTCH1, PTCH2, SMO or SUFU proteins. PTCH1 gene mutations prevent PTCH1 protein from binding to

SMO. Unbound SMO allows unregulated cell growth through activation of the following: transcription factors (proteins that bind to specific DNA sequences and control the flow of genetic information from DNA to RNA) GLI1 (glioma-associated oncogene 1; also called zinc finger protein) and GLI2 cell proliferation genes (cyclin D, cyclin E, myc), and regulators of the process involving the growth of new blood vessels (angiogenesis) [27].

Increasing BCC risk arises from mutations in the PTCH1, PTCH2, SMO and SUFU genes predispose patients to BCC. Up to 70 % of people with sporadic BCC without Gorlin syndrome have patched PTCH1 gene mutations as a result of UV radiation exposure. In 10–20 % of patients with sporadic BCC, mutations in the SMO gene allow for unregulated signaling of tumor growth. A small number of sporadic BCC patients have mutations in the PTCH1 homologue PTCH2 (a variant of the PTCH1 gene) and in the suppressor of fused (SUFU) gene. Patients with Gorlin syndrome are born with an inherited mutation of one allele of the PTCH1 gene. This leads to an autosomal dominant syndrome of cancer predisposition. The remaining good allele can undergo mutation through UV radiation exposure in one lifetime, such that these patients can develop BCC tumors at an earlier age than the general population [28].

In addition, here is evidence that mutations in the tumor suppressor gene P53 and the melanocortin-1 receptor gene may be involved in the development of sporadic BCC. The gene P53 encodes the protein P53, which has been termed 'guardian of the genome'. The P53 protein functions to sense genotoxic injury and arrest cell division allowing DNA repair to occur before replication. In the case of extensive DNA damage, it induces apoptosis (cell death) in an effort to eliminate defective and potentially malignant cells. Mutations of P53 occur in a wide variety of human cancers including BCC. In 44–100 % of BCC patients, mutations in the P53 gene are found, most likely as a result of exposure to UV rays. Arsenic exposure is well known to contribute to BCC formation and is thought to occur through DNA methylation of genes in the P53 pathway [29].

The MC1R gene codes for the melanocortin-1 receptor (MC1R) protein expressed on the surface of melanocytes. Upon stimulation by the α-melanocyte-stimulating hormone (αMSH), it leads to production of melanin in the skin and hair. If the MC1R gene is a wild type, eumelanin is produced leading to tanned skin and dark hair. The MC1R red hair color (RHC) variants lead to the production of pheomelanin and the RHC phenotype: fair skin, red hair, freckles and a higher susceptibility to melanoma and non-melanoma skin cancers. Various studies confirm the association of MC1R variants with BCC risk and show that a fair complexion in addition to MC1R variants greatly increases this risk [29].

Mutations/variants of the following genes may predispose patients to sporadic BCC: glutathione-S-transferase gene (cellular glutathione-S-transferases are involved in the protection against oxidative stress on the skin). P 450 CYP enzyme gene (cytochrome P450 enzymes are involved in detoxification of numerous xenobiotics including carcinogenic components of tobacco smoke), DNA repair gene XRCC3, cyclin-dependent kinase inhibitor genes CDKN2A and CDKN2B basal keratinocyte, and keratin K5 gene BRM gene [30].

Vismodegib (trade name Erivedge™) is a hedgehog pathway inhibitor that was approved in 2012 for the treatment of advanced and metastatic BCC. A number of other experimental therapies targeting molecules of the HH signaling pathway are in early stages of investigation and development [30].

Acne

Acne is a very common skin disorder due to the combined actions of androgenic hormone stimulation of sebaceous glands, abnormal and copious amounts of sebum production, infection by Propriobacterium acnes, obstruction of sebaceous ducts, inflammatory responses, diet and genetics resulting in the formation of plugged pores (comedones) and lesions known commonly as "pimples." Family and twin studies reveal acne aggregates within families with first-degree relatives of acne sufferers having a three to fourfold increased risk of acne.

Acne vulgaris is an under-studied common genetic disease with tremendous economic consequences. Acne vulgaris is one of the most common skin conditions treated by doctors. It affects 40–50 million people in the USA, with prevalence as high as 85 %. Predisposition to acne manifestations is likely polygenic with polymorphisms in CYP1A1, CYP21, TNF-alpha, PEM and IL-1 alpha [31].

Duke University is currently involved in a study "Identifying the Genetic Predictors of Severe Acne Vulgaris and the Outcome of Oral Isotretinoin Treatment" Outcome measures include therapeutic response to isotretinoin and adverse events. All 250 patients with severe acne will be genotyped using the Illumina 610 BeadChip. Whole-exome sequencing will be performed on 100 extremely severe acne vulgaris patients, selected based on severity and response to oral isotretinoin treatment. Given the frequency and severity of severe acne, the predictable severe toxicity of systemic retinoid therapy, and the already demonstrated genetic associations found in Mendelian forms of severe acne, it seems likely that significant genetic risk factors may be identified in patients with severe acne which would promote new and safer therapy, including dietary adjustment [31].

In 2002, Cordain et.al., published an article titled "Acne vulgaris: A Disease of Western Civilzation" wherein they reported "the prevalence of acne in two nonwesternized populations: the Kitavan Islanders of Papua New Guinea and the Aché hunter-gatherers of Paraguay. Additionally, they analyzed how elements in nonwesternized environments may influence the development of acne. Observations of 1200 Kitavan subjects examined (including 300 aged 15–25 years); no case of acne (grade 1 with multiple comedones or grades 2–4) was observed. Of 115 Aché subjects examined (including 15 aged 15–25 years) over 843 days, no case of active acne (grades 1–4) was observed. Further, Cordain described the diets of the Kitavan Islanders as: "Tubers, fruit, fish, and coconut represent the dietary mainstays in Kitava. Virtually all of the dietary carbohydrate intake was in the form of low–glycemic load tubers, fruits, and vegetables" and the diets of the Aché hunter-gatherers as: "cultigens, wild game, small amounts of Western foods, domestic meat, and collected forest products. The cultigens consisted mainly of sweet manioc, followed by peanuts, maize, and rice, whereas the Western goods are mainly pasta, flour, sugar, yerba tea, and bread" [32].

Nutrigenomics

Nutrigenomics is the study of how nutrients influence an individual's genome. This influence encompasses dietary effect at the level of the gene, the protein, and the metabolite. Individual genetic makeup leads to different nutrients having diverging effects at the individual level. Additionally, much like drugs, the therapeutic and toxicity level of nutrients can vary in individuals, along with the point at which someone will be deficient in a nutrient, all according to their individual needs. With the following examples of nutrient effect on genome, keep in mind these aforementioned considerations.

Nutrigenomics builds on these three "omics" disciplines: Transcriptomics, Proteomics, and Metabolomics. As advances in nutrigenomics occur, the prediction of Cordain et al, "that it is possible that low–glycemic load diets may have therapeutic potential in reducing symptoms of acne, a disease virtually unknown to the Aché and Kitavans, may become a reality" [32].

Nutrition at the Gene Interface

Nutrients are involved in various metabolic reactions. These include transcription factor ligands such as the plant based nutrient genistein [33] which has been shown to inhibit an epidermal growth factor receptor and shown promise for alleviating some symptoms of menopause [34], or the plant based nutrient resveratrol which inhibits a TGF-beta pathway [35] and has shown some evidence toward negating aging, carcinogenesis, inflammation, and oxidation. This has been postulated to have consequences for improvement of chronic disease or even aiding in life longevity [36].

Nutrition in DNA Integrity

Genomic integrity is another mechanism in which nutrition plays a role. Prevention of DNA damage has long been associated with anti-oxidant foods. Specifically these encompass nutrients such as folate, B12, niacin, vitamin E, retinol, and calcium. Likewise, some nutrients have been shown with excessive amounts to result in DNA damage, such as riboflavin, pantothenic acid, and biotin [37]. This is dependent on a person's genome, but serves as a key example of the value of nutrigenomics.

Genome Interactions with Nutritional, Economic, and Cultural Factors

As an avid student of medical anthropology and public health (RAN), I have read dozens of articles and books on how cultural problems and access to care issues influence our health. And as a clinician for more than three decades, I have seen first-hand how cultural boundaries and limited health care create medical havoc. Countless dermatologists have witnessed patients who finally got health insurance come in to see them with enormous skin cancers or horrible psoriasis. We can develop very sophisticated genetic research and treatment tools but may be limited by a number of cultural and economic factors.

At the Department of Molecular and Cellular Biology at the University of California, Davis, Raymond Rodriguez directs a unique program. He is the Director and Professor at the Center of Excellence for Nutritional Genomics Department of Molecular & Cellular Biology.

Per the center's web site, "The mission of the Center is to reduce and ultimately eliminate health disparities resulting from adverse environment x genome interactions, particularly those involving nutritional, economic, and cultural factors. Our goal is to devise evidence-based nutritional interventions to prevent, mitigate and delay the onset of diseases such as obesity, Type 2 diabetes, cardiovascular disease, malnutrition and certain cancers." More description is included about achieving this goal by "taking an interdisciplinary approach to develop culturally compatible methods and novel technologies to elucidate the complex interactions between environmental triggers, genes, and disease" [38].

The Center uses a multidisciplinary approach to investigate the influence of diet and individual genetic variation as risk factors for health disparities in racial/ethnic populations in the United States. As stated, "Certain genotypes are more severely affected by specific types of dietary factors than other genotypes, though no genotype is completely immune to the deleterious effects of poor diet." Genomics, proteomics and bioinformatics are used to identify and characterize genes regulated by naturally occurring constituents in foods and those gene-subsets that influence the balance between health and disease. The site states, "Such knowledge is necessary, but not sufficient, to address health disparities among racial/ethnic populations and the poor. Social, economic and cultural factors also come into play when selecting foods and when designing studies to identify causative genes and environmental factors." Hopefully the research at the center and other research facilities will help to improve the care of the skin and its contents [38, 39].

Dermatology: Putting It All Together

Dermatology is a broad field where individuality clearly comes into play. Despite similar structures of proteins, collagen, fibers, nerves, cells, and blood vessels, people display varying reactions in their skin. Some people get cystic acne vulgaris, others clear skin for all of their life. Some may get terrible burns from the sun, others deep tans. Some may get a melanoma that encroaches aggressively on their internal system, others an in-situ carcinoma that responds well to treatment. Some of these variations are hereditary, others acquired, and many idiopathic. Personalized nutrition offers an exciting opportunity to work with the individualized nature of dermatological pathologies.

Nutrigenetics offers the chance to work with the eczema related to food allergies that are innate to an individual genetic makeup. It allows physicians to counteract metabolic disorders such as in PKU with avoiding dietary phenylalanine to prevent the dermatological, neurological, and developmental manifestations, or even avoid internal-medicine related conditions such as the dermatitis herpetiformis of celiac disease by going gluten free.

Nutrigenomics offers a chance to fight various malignancies with attention to structural integrity of the genome, especially in the face of genetic susceptibility. This is where the two principles of personalized nutrition can come together. Also, the involvement of key nutrients that have influence on both chronic disease and aging have significant implications for the field of dermatology. Psoriasis, eczema, and lupus all have chronic components that could benefit from such a study. The cosmetic area of dermatology could make positive changes with new information on ways to slow the process of aging. There are many avenues in this discipline for personalized nutrition to follow. The popular and medical literature is filled with hundreds of books, articles, and stories detailing how certain diets and external applications can benefit the skin, but detailed scientific studies must be done to prove their validity.

Over the last several years in our practice (RAN) we have incorporated oral swabs into selected parts of our diagnostic regimens to help detect which of a patient's current medications are effective and also supply the patient with an overview of general susceptibility to cardiac, Alzheimers, and other diseases. We are performing specific research experiments to use various testing methods including skin biopsies and oral swabs to predict the onset of Alzheimers to allow for an earlier initiation of treatment. A further enhancement of these tests would incorporate an analysis of the efficiency of personalized metabolism of various food sources, especially in patients with known family history of particular genetic abnormalities.

Conclusion

As the science concerning genetics is increasing in the field of nutrition, it is opening up exciting opportunities and avenues for research and consumer focused intervention. There is now considerable evidence of the delicate interplay of individual genomes and nutrition. While we have always been aware of the basic aspects of nutrigenetics and nutrigenomics, there is a full swing movement into actual application of these fields. As these fields continue to grow, it is becoming more valuable for individual consumers to get information on their personal genetic code. This code not only provides valuable data on how their genetics will be influenced by nutritional intervention, it can also serve as a framework for which nutritional impacts can be studied. Humans are very different from one another, and it would be exciting if this field of study could elucidate the differences further than what current data has revealed.

Challenges do exist, however, as they will for any substantial endeavor. We have to carefully investigate the synergies of genetics and environment and how they contribute to pathology. The relationship between diet and gene is very complex and we must be aware of ethical issues in prediction and treatment. As we further study the correlation of nutrition, genetics, and skin, it will be exciting to see how deep we can go and what we can uncover.

Another challenge will be the method of study. Currently the likely form will be observational studies or retrospective analysis depending on cost, tools, and availability of subjects. Nevertheless, it is a step in the right direction to highlight this avenue of research in order to make strides in chronic diseases and genetic conditions that otherwise are at a stand-still in management. Conditions such as eczema, psoriasis, or even melasma could be handled differently and more efficiently. Many conditions where we currently offer temporary, repetitive treatments can be re-evaluated with this new perspective, and possibly actual cures can be discovered.

References

1. Genomics and World Health: Report of the Advisory Committee on Health research. Geneva: WHO; 2002.
2. WHA 57.13: Genomics and World Health. Fifty seventh world health assembly resolution, 22 May 2004.
3. Subbiah MTR. http://www.jcadonline.com/2010/11/application-of-nutrigenomics-in-skin--health-nutraceutical-or-cosmeceutical/. Radnitz C, Beezhold B, Dimatteo J. Investigation of lifestyle choices of individuals following a Vegan diet for health and ethical reasons. Appetite. 2015;31:31–6.
4. Subbiah MTR. Understanding the nutrigenomic definitions and concepts at the food-genome junction. Omics J Integr Biol. 2008;12:1–7. Liakou AI, Theodorakis MJ, Zouboulis CC. Nutritional clinical studies in dermatology. Nutrition and skin. J Drugs Dermatol. 2013;10:209–20.
5. El-Sohemy A. Nutrigenetics. Forum Nut. 2007;60:25–30.
6. Mead MN. Nutrigenomics: the genome–food interface. Environ Health Perspect. 2007;115:A582–9.
7. What are Single Nucleotide Polymorphisms (SNPs)? Genetics home reference http://ghr.nlm.nih.gov/handbook/genomicresearch/snp.
8. James SJ, Melnyk S, Pogribna M, Pogribny IP, Caudill MA. Elevation in S-adenosylhomocysteine and DNA hypomethylation: potential epigenetic mechanism for homocysteine-related pathology. J Nut. 2002;132:2361S–6.
9. Gaboon NE. Nutritional genomics and personalized diet. Egy J Med Hum Genet. 2011;12:1–7.
10. Sloan AE, Powers ME. A perspective on popular perceptions of adverse reactions to foods. J Allergy Clin Immunol. 1986;78(1 Pt 2):127–33.

11. Sicherer S, Sampson HA, eds. Food allergies. Practice essentials, background, pathophysiology. 2009. doi:http://dx.doi.org/10.1016/j.jaci.2009.08.028.
12. Kumar V, Wijmenga C. Celiac disease: update from the 14th International Celiac Disease Symposium 2011. Expert Rev Gastroenterol Hepatol. 2011;5(6):685–7.
13. Kurppa K, Salminiemi J, Ukkola A, Saavalainen P, Löytynoja K, Laurila K, et al. Utility of the new ESPGHAN criteria for the diagnosis of celiac disease in at-risk groups: a large family-based cohort study. J Pediatr Gastroenterol Nutr. 2012;54(3):387–91.
14. Baron DN, Dent CE, Harris H, Hart EW, Jepson JB. Hereditary pellagra-like skin rash with temporary cerebellar ataxia, constant renal amino-aciduria, and other bizarre biochemical features. Lancet. 1956;271(6940):421–8.
15. Chhabra N, Sahil Chhabra S, editors. Protein metabolism. A case oriented approach towards biochemistry. 1st ed. Louisville: Jaypee Brothers Medical Publishers; 2012. p. 128–9.
16. Williams RA, Mamotte CD, Burnett JR. Phenylketonuria: an inborn error of phenylalanine metabolism. Clin Biochem Rev. 2008;29(1):31–41.
17. Phenylketonuria. Practice essentials, background, pathophysiology. http://emedicine.medscape.com/article/947781-overview#a1.
18. Yannicelli S, Ryan A. Improvements in behaviour and physical manifestations in previously untreated adults with phenylketonuria using a phenylalanine-restricted diet: a national survey. J Inherit Metab Dis. 1995;18(2):131–4.
19. Halder B, Bhattacharya U, Mukhopadhyay S, Giri AK. Molecular mechanism of black tea polyphenols induced apoptosis in human skin cancer cells: involvement of Bax translocation and mitochondria mediated death cascade. Carcinogenesis. 2008;29(1):129–38.
20. Bouzari N, Romagosa Y, Kirsner RS. Green tea prevents skin cancer by two mechanisms. J Invest Dermatol. 2009;129:1054.
21. Black H, et al. Effect of a low-fat diet on the incidence of actinic keratosis. N Engl J Med. 1994;330:1272–5.
22. Chen C, et al. A Phase 3 Randomized Trial of Nicotinamide for Skin-Cancer Chemoprevention. N Engl J Med. 2015;373(17):1618–26. doi: 10.1056/NEJMoa1506197.
23. Vlajinac HD, Adanja BJ, Lazar ZF, et al. Risk factors for basal cell carcinoma. Acta Oncol. 2000;39(5):611–6.
24. Lei U, Masmas TN, Frentz G. Occupational non-melanoma skin cancer. Acta Derm Venereol. 2001;81(6):415–7.
25. Letzel S, Drexler H. Occupationally related tumors in tar refinery workers. J Am Acad Dermatol. 1998;39(5 Pt 1):712–20.
26. De Zwaan SE, Haass NK. Genetics of basal cell carcinoma. Aust J Dermatol. 2010;51(2):81–92.
27. Madan V, Hoban P, Strange RC, et al. Genetics and risk factors for basal cell carcinoma. Br J Dermatol. 2006;154 Suppl 1:5–7.
28. Bale AE, Yu KP. The hedgehog pathway and basal cell carcinomas. Hum Mol Genet. 2001;10(7):757–62.
29. Zhang H, Ping XL, Lee PK, Wu XL, Yao YJ, Zhang MJ, et al. Role of PTCH and p53 genes in early-onset basal cell carcinoma. Am J Pathol. 2001;158(2):381–5.
30. http://www.dermnetnz.org/pathology/bcc-genetics.html.
31. https://clinicaltrials.gov/ct2/show/NCT01727440.
32. Cordain L, Lindeberg S, Hurtado M, Hill K, Eaton SB, Brand-Miller J. Acne vulgaris: a disease of Western civilization. Arch Dermatol. 2002;138(12):1584–90.
33. Kussmann M, Laurent B, Fay LB. Nutrigenomics and personalized nutrition: science and concept. Pers Med. 2008;5(5):447–55.
34. Akiyama T, Ishida J, Nakagawa S, Ogawara H, Watanabe S, Itoh N, Shibuya M, Fukami Y. Genistein, a specific inhibitor of tyrosine-specific protein kinases. J Biol Chem. 1987;262(12):5592–5.
35. Taylor M. Complementary and alternative approaches to menopause. Endocrinol Metab Clin North Am. 2015;44(3):619–48.

36. Xiao Z, Chen C, Meng T, Zhang W, Zhou Q. Resveratrol attenuates renal injury and fibrosis by inhibiting transforming growth factor-β pathway on matrix metalloproteinase 7. Exp Biol Med (Maywood). 2016 ;241(2):140-6. doi: 10.1177/1535370215598401. Epub 2015 Aug 27.
37. Smoliga JM, Bauer JA, Hausenblas HA. Resveratrol and health – a comprehensive review of human clinical trials. Mol Nutr Food Res. 2011;55(8):1129–41.
38. Mead MN. Nutrigenomics: the genome–food interface. Environ Health Perspect. 2007;115(12):A582–9.
39. http://nutrigenomics.ucdavis.edu/?page=Home.

Chapter 9
Ecological Dermatology

Robert A. Norman

Abstract I will attempt to clearly explain how the context of natural history and observation has informed the modern field of ecological dermatology. Included will be a historical perspective on Gilbert White and Robert Willan, ecological descriptions in dermatology, insight into the life that lives upon our skin, and new ways to measure environmental impact and interaction with the skin.

Keywords Natural history • Robert Willan • Gilbert White • Ecological dermatology • Ecology • Dermatology • Demodex folliculorum • Resident • Transient • Flora • Skin

> Adam had 'em.
> "On the antiquity of parasites".
> By repute the oldest poem in the English language.

The Natural History and Antiquities of Selborne was written by the English naturalist and ornithologist Gilbert White of Hampshire, England [1]. First published in 1789, late in Gilbert White's life, by his brother Benjamin. The book has been continuously in print since then, with nearly 300 editions up to 2007. Benjamin compiled a mixture of Gilbert's letters to other naturalists, including Thomas Pennant and Daines Barrington. He also compared phenology observations made by Gilbert White and William Markwick of the first appearances in the year of different animals and plants and attempted to organize observations of natural history more or less systematically by species and group. It was the late 1700s and certain concepts such as migration had not gained purchase in our collective thoughts. Therefore Gilbert White and other naturalist provided a hypothesis that swallows hibernate at the bottom of ponds like frogs and toads.

Up the road in London, another form of natural history observation and chronicling was taking place, this by a clinician scientist named Robert Willan. His major

R.A. Norman, DO, MPH, MBA
Professor, Department of Dermatology, Nova Southeastern Medical School, Ft. Lauderdale, FL, USA

Dermatology Healthcare, 8002 Gunn Highway, Tampa, FL 33626, USA
e-mail: skindrrob@aol.com

R.A. Norman (ed.), *Personalized, Evolutionary, and Ecological Dermatology*,
DOI 10.1007/978-3-319-41088-3_9

dermatology works can be categorized into two groups: an introduction of the first classification of skin diseases, and the correct clinical descriptions of many diseases. Willan's work was based predominantly on morphologic features rather than on the etiologic or pathophysiologic characteristics of a disease. Willan published a four-part work, *Cutaneous Diseases,* between 1798 and 1808 that contained a classification of skin diseases according to the form of their pathologic products. Willan was also the first to recognize the importance of illustrations in the description of skin disorders and to create the first atlas of skin diseases containing color pictures [2, 3]. He is noted for many crucial discoveries, including the differentiating of psoriasis from leprosy. (Although it still took many years for the psoriatic to not suffer the wrongly applied infectious label of the leper and be ostracized from society).

White focused on phenology, the study of periodic plant and animal life cycle events and how these are influenced by seasonal and interannual variations in climate and habitat. I believe Willan, while describing his dermatology patients, included his own types of phenology, and perhaps launched a field of ecological dermatology. Not only did Willan describe the morphology of each disease along with seasonal variations, tease out subtle integumentary characteristics and pattern recognition, he was able to add to his categories such as melancholic and psychosocial issues, "The psoriasis most frequently occurs in persons who may be said to be of a mixed temperament, having some of the characteristics of the sanguineous, combined with other appearances belonging to the melancholic temperament."

Charles Rosenberg describes how his "contextual viewpoint lies in the way disease concepts function as elements in a communication system, as units of intelligibility. And that intelligibility lies at the heart of medicine as a functioning social institution. Communication implies a mutually comprehensible (or seemingly comprehensible) vocabulary; and disease categories and related notions of etiology and pathology are an important part of that vocabulary, allowing patient and practitioner to share a measure of understanding" [4]. In the times after the Black Death and other plagues fueled by miasma etiologies and before forms of registration, statistics and enumeration in medicine and public health that led to specific health policies, a time existed when Willan and White lived and natural descriptions abounded. Of course, there are overlaps in historical culture, appearance and reason; I just recently had a patient who fully believed her newborn had a hemangioma because she ate strawberries during pregnancy.

Using Willan and others as a launching point, new environmental and ecological descriptions emerged. As Barankin and Ting stated, communication in dermatology is based upon the accurate morphological description of cutaneous lesions and "dermatologists have adopted interesting and descriptive terminology to portray dermatoses that are difficult to depict and visualize, including frequently encountered objects in nature and natural phenomena. Many of these descriptions are able to effectively create rich visual imagery, and they are useful aids for learning and recall." Many have stood the test of time such as varicella (chicken pox) described as "dewdrops on a rose petal." And "raindrops" describe the pattern of hypopigmented areas within larger areas of hyperpigmentation associated with arsenic-induced pigmentation. Arsenic exposure often results in pigmentary changes (hyper- and/or hypopigmentation) and multiple punctate keratoses on the palms and soles that may develop into skin cancers. Inorganic arsenical exposure comes from agricultural, environmental (well water), industrial (glass workers, miners), and medicinal (herbal) remedies. "Footprints in the snow" depicts a diffuse pattern of scarring alopecia on the scalp. A "dry river bed" was often used to describe the appearance of generalized scales on the body in lamellar ichthyosis and very thick scales referred to as an "armor plate," perhaps observed in an armadillo or turtle. An "ash-leaf" spot is commonly used to describe the shape of lance-ovate hypopigmented macules in tuberous sclerosis [5].

After thirty years of gardening the skin, hair and nails, I have become continually obsessed with the bigger questions about our coverings. Many of these questions include: Why is our skin considered our outer brain? What was our original first color and why did our colors change? What will happen to our skin in the future?

On the more adventurous side: Why are we not still the hairy beasts of old? Why do we have pubic hair? What happened to our claws? Which other beings have nails?

Think of the terrain of the skin and the underlying connections. Why is the skin so connected to the nervous system? The skin, in common with the nervous system, arises from the outermost of the three embryonic cell layers, the ectoderm, which is the general surface covering of the embryonic body. The central nervous system's primary function is keeping the organism informed of what is going on outside it. It develops as the in-turned portion of the general surface of the embryonic body. The rest of the surface covering, after the differentiation of the brain, spinal cord, and all the other parts of the central nervous system, becomes the skin and its derivatives—hair, nails, and teeth. The ectoderm also gives rise to the sense organs of smell, taste, hearing, vision, and touch—everything involved with what goes on outside. Thus, one might consider the nervous system a buried part of the skin, and the skin might be regarded as the external nervous system. These two organ systems begin in intimate association and remain interconnected throughout life. As Frederic Wood Jones, the early twentieth-century English anatomist, put it, "He is the wise physician and philosopher who realizes that in regarding the external appearance of his fellow men he is studying the external nervous system and not merely the skin and its appendages."

We are simply one of over two million species of animals and plants. And like our fellow mortal inhabitants, we are at the mercy of the tiny virus, bacterium, or yeast. Our skin accounts for approximately 16 % of our total body weight and varies in thickness from one millimeter on the eyelids to three millimeters between the shoulder blades and on the palms and soles. People who habitually go barefoot may have soles 1 cm thick. Each of us has about as many bacteria and yeasts on the surface of his or her skin as there are people on earth. The life that lives upon us not only puts our lives in perspective but also allows us a peek at a world within the worlds of our integument, perhaps strange to fathom, yet amazing.

Excuse the pun, but it is all a question of scale. Fleas have parasites. Bacteria can parasitize the parasites of fleas. Viruses can parasitize the same bacteria. As Jonathan Swift put it:

> So naturalists observe, a flea
> Hath smaller fleas that on him prey:

And these have smaller fleas to bite'em,
And so proceed ad infinitum

Yeasts and fungi are inhabitants of the human skin. A yeast is a single-celled fungus which reproduces by budding. The daughter cell grows out from the parent and eventually breaks free. Pityrosporum, which belongs to the family Cryptococcaceae, is the most common yeast on our skins. The genus Pitrosporum ovale are oval spheres about 2 μm wide and 4 μm long which flourish on our hair and fatty parts of our skin. The scalp and around the nose are prime areas where the Pitrosporum ovale population can total half a million per square centimeter. Pityrosporum orbiculare, a round yeast of about 2 μm, can bring on problems when it turns into another form. Filaments called hyphae expand into a spreading mycelium or root-like growth of fungus.

We have probably all seen patients with yeast infections following the chronic use of steroid creams and ointments. Steroids are helpful to calm the inflammation of diseases such as eczema, but they also can suppress the body's natural immune defenses that sets up yeast for a sumptious feast. Or what if Demodex folliculorum staged a revolution?

What do you think of when you think of mites? The disease-filled Middle Ages? Demodex is as jovial and well-adjusted, if I may be anthropormorphic, on clean hair as on dirty and craves blue blood as much as red. The parasites of the human body, in fact, have shown no respect for social order or class as they have evolved with us through the millennia.

Demodex mites are part of normal human fauna. The mites are in the order Arachnida, along with mites, ticks, spiders, and scorpions. Demodex mites are common commensals of the pilosebaceous unit in mammals. However, there is no consensus to what degree the mites are causative of the skin pathology and how they might contribute to the disease.

Demodex folliculorum usually involves the face and Demodex brevis commonly infests the chest and back. Rosacea, a multiphasic disease, is associated with flushing, erythrosis, papulopustular rosacea and phymas; each phase is likely to have its own treatment. Demodex is important in the inflammatory reaction. Helicobacter pylori has also been associated with rosacea.

In immunocompromised hosts Demodex may overpopulate and bring on a dermatitis. The related follicle mite in dogs is responsible for mange. It appears identical but is unable to live on man. Demodex mites are implicated in demdectic alopecia or "human mange."

Demodex, each a third of a millimeter long, is our constant miniature companion throughout life. Although the effect of their presence is still in dispute, as many as 25 mites have been found hanging on to one human eyelash root, which questions their benignity. Each of their individual movements, due to their size, is below the threshold to sensory perception.

As Michael Andrew writes of Demdodex in his 1977 book *The Life That Lives on Man,* "Nothing amongst all the unsuspected secrets of one's skin is more astonishing than the thought that the roots of one's eyelashes are colonized by mites. Few people can confront with equanimity the idea that worm-like creatures which have been likened to eight-legged crocodiles squirm out their diminutive lives in warm oily lairs in our hair follicles." [6]

> Pull down thy vanity, it is not man
> Made courage, or made order, or made grace,
> Pull down thy vanity, I say pull down.
> Learn of the green world what can be thy place
> In scaled invention or true artistry,
> Pull down thy vanity…
> The green casque has outdone your elegance.
> EZRA POUND (from Canto LXXXI)

What else of our normal flora?

The skin is sterile at birth but only remains so briefly. Examining the umbilicus for S. aureus shows 25 % colonization in the first day of life with a steady increase from then on. We have two types of normal skin flora—transient and resident. Resident flora are capable of multiplication and survival and are found as the dominant component in most skin areas. Resident populations on our skins and cilia (sweeping bristles) in our air passages generally protect us from the incursions of foreign organisms.

Resident flora include propionibacterium acnes, a prototype anaerobic diptheroid, found in large numbers with the sebaceous follicles of the skin in moist areas. The organisms may contribute to the inflammatory component of acne. Corynebacterium maximize in the high moisture areas, and like to congregate in the axilla and interdigital skin of the foot.

In contrast to S. aureus, which is found on only 20 % of people, Staphylococcus epidermis is uniformly present on the normal skin. The huge numbers of this resident flora exerts a suppressive effect on other organisms wishing to colonize.

Anaerobic staphylococci are also constantly present. However, they have population densities well below that of other resident flora and unlike other staphylococci do not increase in numbers in dermatologic disease. Gram-negative organisms such as E. Coli, Proteus, and Enterobacter are uncommon on normal human skin except in moist intertriginous (skin touching skin) areas such as toe webs, axillae, and groins. When skin bacteria breaks down the natural secretions from the sebaceous, sweat, and apocrine glands, body odor occurs. Washing with soap and water helps.

Transient flora act as if they have been deposited from the environment or as fallout from mucous membranes. Aerobic spore formers such as Bacillus, various strep, and Neiseria may briefly visit. Specific ecologic data is difficult to obtain due to sampling data and the transitory changes that occur in each part of our skin.

So-called opportunistic pathogens, bacteria and fungi are generally nonpathogenic members of the resident or transient flora, but can trigger infections in debilitated or compromised hosts. In conditions when the skin is immunocompromised, such as in severe eczema, secondary infection by staph aureus is common.

Skin disease due to S. aureus is the most common of all bacterial infections. Impetigo, with its characteristic yellow crusts and transient vesiculation, and folliculitis, which is a circumscribed infectious process originating in a hair follicle, are generally the most superficial of all staphylococcal skin infections. Tiny red pustules congregate around hair follicles. When the infection is recurrent and chronic in the beard area it is called sycosis barbae. Furunculosis (boils) occurs either from an antecedent folliculitis or as deep-seated nodule around a hair follicle. More than 1.5 million cases of furunculosis (boils) occur annually in the USA alone.

Our tissues are particularly vulnerable to infection in the operating theatre, especially in those patients undergoing extended surgeries such as hip joint replacements. Staphylococcus aureus and other opportunistic bacteria can flourish in a wound with invasion infecting from the patient's own bacteria. However, the primary concern in hospitals is cross-infection by resistant organisms.

Although Leeuwenhoek discovered bacteria, it was two centuries later when Pasteur tied in their existence to disease in Homo sapiens. Incidentally, following his discovery Pasteur suffered from a morbid fear of dirt and infections; he avoided shaking hands for fear of a contamination [7].

Pasteur also help to create the world in which cleanliness was next to godliness, which has evolved into a religious zeal, displayed incessantly on our television screens, how the death of germs and their byproducts by disinfectants, deodorants, sprays, and cleaning chemicals germs became a religion, proselytized nightly on the television at enormous costs. But perhaps with a little knowledge, we may find the presence of germs on skin might not be so terrible.

Although when we envision life on the skin as the creeping and hopping evident in larger creatures, the huge majority of our fellow travelers of our own private zoological gardens, numerically, are harmless or beneficial. Each of us supports billions of creatures; since no one can escape from our animal origins it is wise to understand what is happening. Just as we have only begun to explore the undersea world and outer space, the world of our skin is still a great mystery. Our skin is an ecosystem, just like the rivers and hammocks, and carries with it all the same issues—self-sustaining boundaries, competitive forces for food and growth, and intimate interconnections between itself and resident and transient flora. When a person takes a broad-spectrum antibiotic such as tetracycline, he or she does so with the risk that the diverse set of microclimates of our ecosystem will suffer from imbalance. Our skins have no seasons or diurnal variation and comparatively limited temperature ranges, but has the same complexity and need for ecological integrity of many ecosystems. And given adequate nutrition and care, the skin has tremendous self-healing powers [7].

> All the wise world is little else, in Nature,
> But parasites and sub-parasites.
> Ben Jonson

Every move you make (sounds like a Sting song) results in showers of skin particles released into the air. Every 24 h an estimated 10,000 million skin scales or squames peel off each of our bodies, accounting for one to one-and-a-half grams of skin a day, or about one pound every year. The squames are the desiccated remnants of skin cells that continually form at the base of the epidermis and travel slowly outwards. After 40 to 56 days a newly formed cell reaches the surface. It has died from the formation of keratin fibers, the same horny components of our hair and finger-nails, and is called the stratum corneum. The dead cells are closely attached to each other to form what we call our skin.

At high magnification this surface dead skin appears as irregular patches of curling rough and curly cornflakes. House dust consists of 80–90 % skin; squames are the motes in the sunbeam filtering into our rooms.

Viruses are the smallest live inhabitants of our skins and can only reproduce by entering a living cell and fooling it into making more of their own genetic material. The viruses multiply inside the captive cell until they burst, releasing more virus to colonize other cells. When we have any lowering of our resistance—an infection, sunburn, or stress–the Herpes virus *hominis* which brings on "cold sores" may step into the picture. The virus, which usually begins in childhood, may appear on the skin and then return to the underlying nerves, ebbing and flowing based on the individual's immunity. Once infected, the virus is carried for life, and more than 90 % of the population carry Herpes virus.

Andrews wrote, "Wherever man goes he is not alone. Though we may leave the Earth we take with us on any voyage of discovery our own personal world which is yet to be completely explored. We evolved on Earth, but we did so in the company of the minute creatures which live out their lives on our bodies. We should treat our fellow travelers with respect; they are much more adaptable than we are, and they do us more good than harm."

What of the future? We may have skin detective agencies utilizing bacteriological forensic techniques, pointing to individuals at the scene of a crime. Perhaps the characteristic microflora of a suspect could be just as important to the detective as a fingerprint or other genetic markers. If an individual's microflora, established shortly after birth, remains comparatively constant throughout life, a microbial sampling of room dust, saliva and so on, might reveal groups of identifiable organisms which would match the pattern of a suspect. The particular manner of acquisition of the many different phage-types of bacteria from mother, hospital and early contacts could differentiate two suspects who would support different organisms. By sophisticated phage-typing methods, bacteria could be called to give evidence in court.

Perhaps the old adage about "what you don't see can't hurt you" applies. The huge majority or those critters that live on the skin are invisible and earn our indifference. And when it does bother us, at least we have treatments. As far as I know, we are the only species to have dermatologists, and nail salons, and beauty parlors, and a myriad of other sources to rid our body of real or perceived ailments. I am forever humbled, for along with my fellow soldiers who fight these ever-lasting skin diseases, I know we can never win the battle. We all still choose to fight, to provide momentary solace from the onslaught of our own invaders for the untold numbers of patients we all treat with skin infestations every year, and hopefully provide a little help along the way.

While exploring the internet, I discovered an International Association of Ecodermatology (http://www.skineco.org/) based in Rome, Italy. Part of the mission of the group appears to influence the world of cosmetics by revising cosmetics and assessing their environmental impact and interaction with the skin. Noted is that the degree of cosmetic consumption in Europe has risen substantially, with a yearly average of 2 million tons of cosmetics consumed within the 25 EC countries. Approximately 5,100 t of cosmetic products released into the environment every day and the current European legislation does not as yet take into account the biodegradability of the substances used in cosmetics. The group is attempts to study and develop eco-friendly formulations and support "all the eco-friendly companies that are ready to become ecologically responsible, by analyzing part or all of the product life cycle, from formulation to production, up to skin interaction and final disposal." In addition the members appear to have a goal of measuring, studying and evaluating the effects of climate changes and environmental pollution (air and water) on skin and to develop guidelines for environmental risk management in relation with the skin and for defining an eco-dermo-compatible certification [8].

New discoveries in coming years will hopefully uncover the evolutionary and ecological reasons including genetic markers (when known) for these skin changes related to nature and other species. Most new findings may have delighted White and Willan and others. Had Willan been able to peer into the future, he may have been amazed by the current understanding of what lives on us. In particular, it seems fascinating that as we explore the ecological landscape of the skin, we also describe a disease like psoriasis as a heterogenous and complex disease grouped by endotypes (endophenotypes) defined functionally and pathologically by molecular mechanisms. We classify skin diseases by treatment response and how translational medicine can affect the outcome of care, and will increasingly use ecological dermatology as a springboard for further research and study.

Acknowledgement Thanks to Professor Chris Griffiths from Manchester England for his 2015 Society for Investigative Dermatology Eugene Farber lecture "A natural history of psoriasis"

References

1. White G. The natural history and antiquities of Selborne. London: Benjamin White; 1789.
2. Willan R. Cutaneous diseases. Philadelphia: Kimber and Conrad, Brown & Merritt; 1798–1808.
3. Grzybowski A, Parish LC. Robert Willan: pioneer in morphology. Clin Dermatol. 2011;29(2):125–9.
4. Rosenberg C. What is disease? Memory of Owsei Temkin. Bull History Med. 2003;77(3): 491–505.
5. Ting P, Barankin B. Environmental terminology in the language of dermatology. Division of Dermatology and Cutaneous Sciences. University of Alberta, Edmonton
6. Andrews M. The life that lives on man. New York: Taplinger; 1977.
7. Norman R. The Blue Man and other stories of the skin. Berkeley: University of California Press; 2014.
8. International Association of Ecodermatology. http://www.skineco.org/

Chapter 10
Skin Color

Robert A. Norman

Abstract Caring for skin of color is a field of dermatology that is becoming increasingly important. Improving our understanding of the nuances of skin color allows practitioners to have more precision with their treatments, and provides more specific photo-protection techniques and personalized treatment options. Here I will provide an overview of skin color including the evolution of skin color, tanning, and the cultural implications of skin color.

Keywords Genetics • Skin • Skin cancer • Skin color • Melanosomes • Tanning • Bleaching • Albinism • Vitiligo • Jamaica • Haiti • Medical Anthropology

The Melanocyte and Tanning

Why does our skin get darker over time and exposure to the sun? The main reason is the oxidative stress placed on melanin as it performs the reactions with ultraviolet light, protecting us from dangerous rays.

Melanocytes live in the bottom layer of the epidermis above the dermis and manufacture melanin from an amino acid, tyrosin, with the help of an enzyme, tyrosinase. Exposures of 5–10 min of sunshine do not bring on tan, but longer than that will cause the initiation of a process called melanogenesis. UV light stimulates the production of melanin in the form of insoluble melanosomes that surround the epidermal cells, which move up to the surface of the skin and result in a tan.

Many societies today value the appearance of a dark tan, causing many people to expose themselves to high levels of UV radiation. No safe tan exists; it is another form of burn.

Kurt Vonnegut was asked to be the guest speaker for a prestigious college's commencement eercise, and this is the first and last portion of what he told the graduating

R.A. Norman, DO, MPH, MBA
Dermatology Healthcare, 8002 Gunn Highway, Tampa, FL 33626, USA

Professor, Department of Dermatology, Nova Southeastern Medical School, Ft. Lauderdale, FL, USA
e-mail: skindrrob@aol.com

R.A. Norman (ed.), *Personalized, Evolutionary, and Ecological Dermatology*,
DOI 10.1007/978-3-319-41088-3_10

class. "Wear sunscreen. If could offer you only one tip for the future, sunscreen would be it. The long-term benefits of sunscreen have been proved by scientists, whereas the rest of my advice has no basis more reliable than my own meandering experience…Advice is a form of nostalgia. Dispensing it is a way of fishing the past from the disposal, wiping it off, painting over the ugly parts and recycling it for more than it's worth. But trust me on the sunscreen."

During my childhood summers in Michigan, where I grew up a distance less than an hour from the beach, I had cherished the sun. I recall the smell of baby oil mixed in with the thin toasty smell of heated skin. I savored the precious two months of the year when I could actually lay in the sun with scant clothing, the memories of giant snow piles melting to my mind's periphery. Now, as an adult I had to worry about what I had thought of as a benevolent sun being some type of malicious nuclear reactor that had melted down my skin and turned my DNA into a skin cancer-making machine. I need to add eternal vigilance about the devastating effects of the sun to all the other problems of our day-to-day life—the threat of terrorism, Lyme disease, West Nile virus and long lines at Starbucks. And, as a dermatologist, I have to help others heed the wake-up call.

The first Greek sun god was Helios. We use the term dermatoheliosis in reference to photoaging or sun damage on the skin. Later Apollo became the accepted sun god. Apollo was also the god of healing and prophecy. Aesculapius, Apollo's mortal son, was said to be the first physician, and his staff entwined by a serpent is Western medicine's symbol. Over 400 years ago, Copernicus declared the sun as the center of our universe. The healing power of the sun has always been evident, from cave dwellers worshiping the sun to the sun's germicidal powers and ability to diminish various skin diseases such as psoriasis. Vitamin D synthesis and the feel-good effects of the sun (an antidote to seasonal affective disorder for those in dreary Northern climates) also play major sun roles. But perhaps not even Apollo could foresee the sun's damaging effects on future generations [1]

How did this oceanic change in our sense of the sun come about? Much of the history of sun tanning carries with it a media hype akin to cigarette smoking. During the 1920s and 1930s, many movie stars were paid to smoke at peak attention-getting locations, thus enabling the tobacco companies to increase their sales dramatically. In similar fashion, the Coco Chanels of the world launched huge media and tanning spikes. Betty Grable, Rita Hayworth, and other bathing beauties were pictured in one and two-piece bathing suits exposing their tan bodies.

European women sun bathed in decorative, attention-getting sun hats and shawls for fashionable reasons, not protection. And if their skin happened to have any spot without a tan, brown and beige tinted powders and creams were available. The fashion world created shoes to be worn without stockings and sleeveless dresses for women wishing to expose their tans. And a tan in the winter was a clear sign that the tan bearer had enough wealth and leisure to afford an exotic, warm climate.

In 1929 Helena Reubenstein warned, "Sun burn menaces your beauty." Women's magazines pushed tanning. Cosmetic companies introduced sun-tanning oils; the ingredient PABA was introduced in 1943. While the public ambiguity about the pale or tanned look persisted, women's magazines encouraged sun lamps and tanning and cosmetic companies introduced sun-tanning oils. The first self-tanning product, Man-Tan, hit the market, with beige, brown, or orange tint results. Certain science reporters used women's magazines to suggest that gradual tanning could cancel out the sun's harmful skin damaging effects. The media slowly took in the message of the sun and the skin. Harper's Bazaar, in 1954, reported, "There are sunscreen preparations that can cut the intensity of the sun's rays by 75 %." In my medical practice, there is not a week that goes by when someone does not say to me, "We didn't know about the problem with the sun when we were younger". They clearly may not have known about it, but it was evident in the media.

Dark skin became a status symbol in the 1960s. Sun tanning was not a spectator sport, especially among the young. Coppertone advertisements filled the airways—"Tan, don't burn, Get a Coppertone tan!" and beach movies filled with bikini-clad teens populated the television. In the 1970s, with gallons of Johnson's baby oil coating many an unsuspecting epidermis, another industry began to blossom–the indoor tanning industry. Even those in the cold North could try and keep a tan or prepare for adventures to warmer climates with a series of trips to the tanning salon. Although ivory skin was once associated with wealth and not working in the fields, this shifted with the rise of the industrial society. Tan skin represented someone who had leisure time. The Hawaiian Tropic TV ad featured a beautiful blonde who sensually said, "White is for laundry."

In the early 1970s the FDA began to treat sunscreens as over-the-counter drugs and not cosmetics. More stringent labeling was required. After the FDA began regulating sunscreens, the makers of Johnson's Baby Oil warned that the heroine of their ads should "take a little less sun." The FDA in 1978 declared sunscreens to be safe, effective, and useful to prevent skin cancer and sunburn and slow down premature aging of the skin. The SPF numbering system was developed using numbers 2–15.

In addition to the cancer-producing and premature wrinkling effects of the sun, home-tanning units emitted high levels of UVB light that burned the skin and didn't tan. More advanced tanning units emitted both UVB and UVA rays and brought on further damage. The tanning industry, almost entirely unregulated, continued to prosper. Keep in mind that ultraviolet radiation (UVR) is responsible for 90 % of the visible signs of aging on the skin of whites.

By the mid-1980s, public education program about the dangers of over exposure to the sun and the problems with self-tanning began to grow. The *American Academy of Dermatology* voiced its strong opinions in support of sun protection, and sunscreen manufacturers produced higher SPF products.

Malignant melanoma studies showed a 500 % increase from 1950 to 1985. A 1987 American Academy of Dermatology study revealed that 96 % of Americans admitted to know that the sun caused skin cancer. One third of the adults in the survey admitted they deliberately worked on a tan.

The indoor tanning industry continued to be one of the fastest growing businesses in America. The average age of the indoor tanning patrons was 26, mostly women. Almost 2 million of these patrons were considered "tanning junkies" with almost 100 tanning parlor visits per year. In 1991, 1800 injuries were reported from tanning devices.

Fashion design industry leaders such as Eileen Ford stated, "The tanned look is dead." The American Academy of Dermatology stated there was "no safe way to tan." following a consensus conference on photo aging and photo damage. (In reality, a tan is simply a controlled burn). And natural-looking tans sans streaking or discoloration were possible with improved tanning products. Wide ranges of protection against UVA as well as UVB radiation were created by the sunscreen industry in 1990 in response to the rising tide of information about skin cancer facts–600,000 new cases of skin cancers, 6300 deaths from melanoma and 2500 deaths from squamous cell carcinoma. The role of genetics, ozone depletion, and other skin cancer production factors took center stage.

The incidence of skin cancer increased, with 700,000 new cases of skin cancer diagnosed in 1993, 32,000 of them malignant melanoma. A survey in 1996 of young adults under 25 indicated 58 % of them confessed to working on a tan and 62 % stated they think people look better with a tan. In 1997, a survey in 17 magazine stated that two thirds of the teens felt they looked better with a tan and felt healthier and more sophisticated. Half of them stated they looked more athletic with a tan. Although more than half the states had rules and regulations for tanning salons, the tanning industry grew to almost 20,000 tanning salons in America with 22 million customers per year. The American Academy of Dermatology continued to warn the public to minimize the sun's damage to the skin and eyes by planning outdoor activities to avoid the sun's strongest rays, wearing protective covering, wearing sunglasses and always wearing a broad spectrum sunscreen.

Why do so many people pound their skin with artificial rays to get a tan? With so many research studies linking UV radiation with skin cancer risks, it might be a good time to close the doors on the Fake n' Bake. According to studies from the American Academy of Dermatology and the U.S. Department of Health & Human Services, tanning increases your risk of melanoma and non-melanoma skin cancer such as squamous cell carcinoma and basal cell carcinoma, and the excessive exposure to UV radiation during indoor tanning leads to skin aging, immune suppression and eye damage, including cataracts and ocular melanoma. Yet more than 1 million people tan in tanning salons on an average day, nearly 70 % of them girls and women aged 16–29.

According to a study by San Diego State University public health researchers published in the American Journal of Preventive Medicine, indoor tanning salons in America's big cities often outnumbered Starbucks or McDonalds? The study looked at the number and density (per 100,000 people) of indoor tanning facilities in 116 of the largest cities in the country and then compared tanning facilities with two "ubiquitous institutions." The city of Charleston, W. Va., took the top prize for the highest density of tanning salons with a total of 18 facilities for a population of more than 53,000, with only one Starbucks and seven McDonald's. Indoor tanning mega-cities included Pittsburgh, Penn, Portland, Maine, Akron, Ohio, and Columbia, South Carolina.

Proximity appears to trump rationality during interviews with 6,000 teens across the country. Living within two miles of a tanning salon increases usage. Sales incentives of monthly discount packages, such as $19 a month for unlimited tanning, and extended hours also bumps up the numbers. Others have promoted "good UVA rays" as opposed to "bad UVB rays," but all data shows and increase in skin cancer and skin aging with the UVA rays from tanning.

Why are so many people still tanning, especially with all the evidence regarding the cumulative effects of UV radiation? Why do we have this mad desire to feed the melanocyte? There are nearly as many answers as there are tanning parlors. According to a 60 min report, by 2013 we will spend 6.6 billion dollars on sun care products.

Some people say they do it for the vitamin D. Indoor tanning and vitamin D replenishment is a myth, because it is safer to eat cheese, drink milk, eat fish or take vitamin supplements. The relaxation or pleasurable feelings that some users report may even be addictive, but exercise is a healthier alternative. For those who suffer from Seasonal Affective Disorder, light boxes can be used even on cloudy winter days that use broad spectrum light, not UV. Others suggest tanning helps with skin problems such as psoriasis, but they should seek environments such as a doctor's office, where the type and dosage of such light is regulated. And for those who feel "healthier" with a bronze tint to their epidermis, there are safe self-tanning lotions and spray-on tans.

Tan-seeking US buyer beware! The Obama administration, to help fund the $940 billion health care overhaul, added a 10 % tax on individuals receiving indoor tanning services, and the initiative is expected to generate $2.7 billion over 10 years.

Although it is has been historically rare to detect skin cancers in African Americans, in my practice I have recently noted an increase in skin cancers in this population. Statistics state that the incidence of skin cancer in blacks is approximately 3 per 100,000 compared to whites, which is 234 per 100,000. The melanin is in greater amounts in the black skin, which protects against ultraviolet radiation and damage to the DNA. The number of melanocytes in blacks and whites is the same, but the way the melanin is distributed and produced is quite different. For both African Americans and whites, the primary risk factor is chronic UVB exposure.

I know it is always difficult to get people to change behavior. Knowing that tanning increases your rate of skin cancer by 75 % may be important–tanning beds are a carcinogen like cigarettes. But the light is also known to increase endorphins, and not everyone wants to run a mile to get the same effect. Many sun protection factor 15 and higher sunscreen were readily available since the early 1980s and, of course, they are available today in a variety of topical preparations. I certainly preach the gospel of using sunscreens, especially to the parents of vulnerable children, which will pay off in huge cost savings and treatment prevention in future years. In a similar fashion, there are patches and pills and other products to quit smoking, but it is difficult. I regularly see patients in their 20s and 30s with skin cancers and have also had a 14- and a 15-year-old in my office presenting with a stage IV malignant melanoma.

The Origins of Skin Color

The most recent scientific evidence indicates that all humans evolved in Africa and then populated the rest of the world through successive generations. It seems likely that the first modern humans had relatively large numbers of eumelanin-producing melanocytes–darker skin–as with the indigenous people of Africa today. As some of these original peoples migrated to areas of Asia and Europe, the selective pressure for eumelanin production decreased in climates where radiation from the sun was less intense.

What other theories have arisen for the etiology of variations in skin color? Some hypotheses include protection from ambient temperature, infections, skin cancer or frostbite, an alteration in food, and sexual selection. Much of the recent research on skin adaptation to the environment involves Vitamin D production. For those who live in northern latitudes, where skin is exposed to meager sunlight, the inhabitants are also unable to make Vitamin D. Vitamin D is necessary to prevent rickets, a bone disease caused by too little calcium. African blacks require intense sunlight to penetrate their dark skin to make Vitamin D. When blacks lived in England during the Industrial Revolution, they were the first to develop symptoms of rickets, with retarded growth, bowed legs and fractures. The theory suggests that at some point northern populations experienced positive selection for lighter skin due to the increased production of vitamin D from sunlight and the genes for darker skin disappeared from these populations. Fortunately, in 1930, Vitamin D was discovered and dispensed as a supplement to add to the diet.

Folate is a key player in the investigation of skin color. Since it is needed for DNA replication in dividing cells, the absence of folate can effect crucial body processes that include the production of sperm cells. Many top researchers, including Professor Nina Jablonski, propose that the ability to produce melanin was selected for in our early human ancestors because it helped preserve the body's supply of folate in addition to reducing the chances of developing skin cancer [2].

The Unbearable Color of Being

Skin bleaching is a widespread problem in the Caribbean, in particular in Jamaica where I do volunteer work and research. Why do people participate in often harmful various techniques of skin lightening? How does the culture and politics play a role in the specific problems of skin bleaching?

One of my personal and research goals is to understand the worldwide, devastating, and growing problem of skin bleaching and issues related to skin color. Like many of my colleagues, I have witnessed the devastating effects of skin bleaching and other skin manipulations over the years.

Skin bleaching (also called skin lightening, skin whitening and skin toning) refers to the practice of using chemical substances to lighten skin tone or provide an even skin complexion by lessening the concentration of melanin. Homemade concoctions, cosmetic products and dermatological products are used to decrease the melanin. Manipulation of skin color has ancient beginnings and the practice continues to grow, often in harmful ways.

Although other personal choices such as tattooing, piercing, or Botox carry inherent risks, skin bleaching is in a whole other and potentially dangerous category. Many of the bleaching mixtures have dangerous components and are purchased form unreliable sources. Major problems occur if bleaching products contain harmful ingredients such as mercury (a metal that blocks production of melanin but also can act as a poison to damage the nervous system), high-potency steroids such as Clobetasol propionate. Improper use of the bleaching products can result in permanent scarring and thinning of the skin. Common problems include uneven color loss, leading to a blotchy appearance and possible blue-black darkening of the skin, permanent skin bleaching, and redness and intense irritation.

The bleaching products are often available for sale over the internet, providing unlimited access to potential customers. According to recent data, in Mali, Nigeria, Senegal, South Africa and Togo, 25 %, 77 %, 27 %, 35 % and 59 % of women, respectively, are reported to use skin lightening products on a regular basis. In 2004, nearly 40 % of women surveyed in China, Malaysia, the Philippines and the Republic of Korea reported using skin lighteners.

Carolyn Cooper, a professor of literary and cultural studies at the University of the West Indies, wrote in The Jamaica Gleaner newspaper, "If we really want to control the spread of the skin-bleaching virus, we first have to admit that there is an epidemic of color prejudice in our society." Certain sociologists and other observers highlight issues such as societies that continue to privilege Whiteness, betraying one's culture, lack of education, media brainwashing, and "colonial mentality."

Professor Christopher Charles, a faculty member of The University of the West Indies, Mona, Jamaica, who has studied the psychology of bleaching wrote that many young Jamaicans perceive it "as a modern thing, like Botox, to fashion their own body in a unique way." Charles writes about the issues of self-hate, self-esteem and the multifactorial reasons behind skin bleaching.

Is there safe use of bleaching creams? Conventional and historic use of bleaching creams containing hydroquinone at 2.0–5.0 % concentrations are modestly effective in treating certain pigmentary disorders. Achieving success depends on diligent, long-term treatment by patients who have carefully instructed in methods of use as well as protection from sun exposure and knowing the signs of allergic contact dermatitis. In Japan, the European Union, and Australia, hydroquinone has been removed from over-the-counter skin products and substituted with other chemicals due to concerns about health risks. In the United States over-the-counter creams containing up to 2 % hydroquinone are recognized to be safe and effective by the U.S. Food and Drug Administration. If low-potency topical corticosteroids, mild salicylic acid, or tretinoin are added under a physician's supervision, improved may occur, although most people experience at best only partial improvement and want more results. The problem is that many people want more demonstrable results in a quicker time and choose high-dose and destructive skin bleaching.

Is there a viable way to decrease the harmful activity of skin bleaching in the Caribbean and throughout the world? In the context of political-economic shifts in the Caribbean, how does political economy and media influence decision-making and skin color choice?

Eva Lewis-Fuller, Jamaican Ministry of Health director of health promotion and protection, states she is redoubling education programs to combat bleaching in this predominantly black island of 2.8 million peoples. Images of fair-skinned people predominate in commercials for high-end products and in the social pages of newspapers. “Bleaching has gotten far worse and widespread in recent years,” Lewis-Fuller said. “(Bleachers) want to be accepted within their circle of society. They want to be attractive to the opposite sex. They want career opportunities. But we are saying there are side effects and risks. It can disfigure your face.”

Campaigns by health officials on local radio stations warn of bleaching hazards, and other efforts have included putting up posters in schools, holding talks and handing out literature about the dangers. A similar anti-bleaching campaign in 2007 called “Don’t Kill the Skin” did little to slow the craze. Although little data exists on the prevalence of damage caused by skin-bleaching agents, dermatologists and other health officials are reportedly seeing more cases.

Evelyn Nakano Glenn, a professor of gender and women’s studies at the University of California, Berkeley and president of the American Sociological Association, has stated it is wrong to assume that skin-lightening was a cultural anachronism or an effort to negate one’s racial heritage. She is quoted in the New York Times as saying, “In fact, it’s a growing practice and one that has been stimulated by the companies that produce these products. Their advertisements connect happiness and success and romance with being lighter skinned.” Glenn denies that dark-skinned women are imagining a bias, and that “Sociological studies have shown among African-Americans and also Latinos, there’s a clear connection between skin color and socioeconomic status. It’s not some fantasy. There is prejudice against dark-skinned people, especially women in the so-called marriage market.”

Comments attributed to the Senate majority leader, Harry Reid, Democrat of Nevada, as reported in a new book, stated that he had urged Barack Obama to run for president because the country was ready to accept a “light skinned” African-American. Many users seek to lighten their entire face or large swatches of their body, as a way to elevate one’s social standing, especially in developing countries such as Senegal, India and the Philippines.

Skin bleaching is a dynamic and compelling problem that requires immediate research and intervention with users to prevent progressive physical and psychological damage. New research and understanding will contribute to public policy. Questions about identity and race, economics, and a holistic approach to a disturbing problem are at the core of the skin bleaching problem. With more discussion, education, and intervention, the problem can be minimized.

Vitiligo and Albinism

Two of the diseases of the skin that involve irregularity in pigmentation are vitiligo and albinism. Vitiligo is due to the absence of one of our main skin characters—the melanocytes–and results in an acquired hypopigmentation. A positive family history exists in at least 30 % of vitiligo patients, and both sexes are affected equally.

About half of the people who develop this skin disorder experience some pigment loss before the age of 20. Even though most people with vitiligo are in good general health, they face a greater risk of having hyperthyroidism or hypothyroidism (increased or decreased thyroid function), pernicious anemia (vitamin B12 deficiency), Addison's disease (decreased adrenal function), alopecia areata (round patches of hair loss), and/or uveitis (inflammation of the eyes).

Whenever I have a patient with vitiligo, it makes me think about our skin color and the many factors that determine our destiny. The skin is the most visible aspect of our appearance, and we have a wide variety of genetically determined skin colors. The melanocyte, a tiny structure, is one of the most important parts of the human body for many reasons, including skin color, sun protection, and cultural determination. Many skin diseases can engender heavy loads of social and psychological stress, but those with pigmentary alterations are often the most devastating. We have racial discrimination, wars, and other haunting acts of violence and evil in society prompted by perceptions about skin color.

The melanocyte provides energy, protection, and the color of our skin and eyes. Melanocytes live in the top layer of the skin and create melanin, which is a widely available substance in nature, even seen in plants and fish. The primary role of melanin in the human body is to act as a natural sun block, absorbing ultraviolet radiation from the sun and quickly converting it into harmless heat. How effective is melanin as a photoprotectant? The photochemical properties of melanin transforms the harmful UV energy via "ultrafast internal conversion" and enables melanin to dissipate more than 99.9 % of the absorbed UV radiation and prevents the indirect DNA damage that is responsible for the formation of malignant melanoma and other skin cancers.

How does melanin and skin color work? Imagine you had a genetic paintbrush and you could mix the colors together, but you only had two colors–pheomelanin (red) and eumelanin (very dark brown). You make your choices on the quantity and type of melanin given, determined by a handful of genes. One copy of each of these genes is inherited from each of our parents and each gene comes in several different versions known as alleles. People with dark skin need more melanin pigment compared to light skinned persons. Differences in the number, size and nature of pigment cells, containing pigment granules called melanosomes, determine the many different shades of skin color. Europeans have fewer, smaller and lighter melanosomes than those from people of West Africa.

Vitiligo affects 1–4 % of the world population, and since ancient times patients with vitiligo have suffered the same mental abuses as lepers. Vitiligo was referred to as *Sweta Kustha* in India, meaning "White leprosy". Although vitiligo is disfiguring in all races, it is particularly true in dark skinned people due to the strong contrast.

Davinder Parsad and other researchers carried out several research projects on the psychosocial implications of pigmentary disorders in Asia. In India, those with vitiligo face severe psychological and social problems, and it is particularly acute in the case of young women and children. The first prime minister of India, Jawaharlal Nehru, ranked vitiligo (commonly known as leucoderma) as one of three major medical problems of India behind leprosy and malaria.

How is vitiligo associated with Indian life and religious beliefs? According to certain Indian religious texts regarding reincarnation a person with vitiligo in this life did "Guru Droh" (sin) in his previous life. Because of the incidence of arranged marriages, vitiligo is particularly debilitating among young unmarried women, who have a slim opportunity for marriage due to the disease. If a married women develops vitiligo, the marriage may end in divorce.

The word "albinism" refers to a group of inherited conditions. People with albinism have little or no pigment in their eyes, skin, or hair; they have inherited albinism genes from both parents that do not make the usual amounts of a pigment called melanin. The exception is one type of ocular albinism, which is passed on from mothers to their sons.

One person in 17,000 in the U.S.A. has some type of albinism. Albinism affects people from all races. Most children with albinism are born to parents who have normal hair and eye color for their ethnic backgrounds. Often people do not recognize that they have albinism.

In less pigmented types of oculocutaneous albinism, (the type of albinism that affects both the skin and the eyes), hair and skin are cream-colored. In types with slight pigmentation, hair appears more yellow or red-tinged. People with ocular albinism (albinism that only affects the eyes) usually have normal or only slightly lighter than normal physical appearance.

Albinism was noted in the earliest medical literature. Several Greek and Roman authors (including Plinius Secundus the elder and Aulus Gellius) described albinism in man. Tyrosinase deficiency in animals was first demonstrated in 1904, and the first accurate scientific paper written about albinism was by Sir Archibald Garrod in 1908.

One of my patients with albinism had grown up in South Africa. "I'm new to this country," he said. "Things were not good where I came from. Because of my skin people there thought I was evil." We had discussed his history and he revealed he had been kept out of school and almost totally ostracized in his community because of his condition. Over the following weeks I did much work to eliminate his skin cancers as I listened to his stories.

The striking appearance of albinism has fascinated humankind for centuries, drawing reactions ranging from veneration to alienation. In some Asian societies dating back to ancient times, and in Europe during the Middle Ages and the Renaissance, fair skin was considered very attractive, a sign of wealth and high social status. Tanned skin meant that one was obligated to work in the fields for one's livelihood. Similarly, the powdered white wig worn by American colonial era illuminati reflected the wearer's ability to afford luxury items and be identified as one of the educated elite.

Nevertheless, in nineteenth-century America, albinism was considered such a bizarre trait that people with this condition were exhibited in circus sideshows. Furthermore, with the advent of the camera, these individuals were featured on postcards, which were widely distributed and collected from the 1870s–1890s. Photo studios such as those of Charles Eisenmann, Obermuller & Son, and Matthew Brady specialized in taking pictures of what were regarded as human oddities.

Many Native American and South Pacific tribes believed that human beings and animals with albinism were messengers from divine entities. Some saw them as good omens and treated them with utmost respect. Others viewed their presence as a manifestation of wrongdoings within the tribe. In Africa, life has always been particularly difficult for people with albinism. Widespread poverty and ignorance about the condition deprives these individuals of much-needed protection from the burning sun. As a result, many die prematurely from skin cancer. Even if they do manage to avoid the strong sunlight, it often means a life of virtual solitary confinement and prohibition from participating in the daily activities of their kinship group.

Even today, a plethora of misconceptions about albinism persists. Bizarre characters (usually villains) labeled "albinos" with snow-white skin and hair, blood-red eyes, and supernatural powers plague the entertainment industry. Many people with albinism have been institutionalized and/or stripped of educational and vocational opportunities due to a misguided belief that the low vision accompanying the condition (on average, 20/200) prevents one from being able to adequately function in and contribute to society. Some members of the medical profession have even been known to recommend abortions to mothers carrying babies with albinism because it was thought that their children would die at an early age and would fail to lead productive lives.

Vision problems in albinism result from abnormal development of the retina and abnormal patterns of nerve connections between the eye and the brain. These eye problems result from abnormal development of the eye because of lack of pigment. The retina, the surface inside the eye that receives light, does not develop normally before birth and in infancy. The nerve signals from the retina to the brain do not follow the usual nerve routes. The iris, the colored area in the center of the eye, lacks sufficient pigment to screen out stray light coming into the eye. (Light normally enters the eye only through the pupil, the dark opening in the center of the iris, but in albinism light can pass through the iris as well.) It is the presence of these eye problems that defines the diagnosis of albinism. The main test for albinism is simply an eye exam.

In the United States, people with albinism live normal life spans and have the same types of general medical problems as the rest of the population. Those who do not use skin protection may develop life-threatening skin cancers. If they use appropriate skin protection, such as sunscreen lotions rated 20 or higher, and opaque clothing, people with albinism can enjoy outdoor activities even in summer.

People with albinism are at risk of isolation, because the condition is often misunderstood. Social stigmatization can occur, especially within communities of color, where the race or paternity of a person with albinism may be questioned. Families and schools must make an effort not to exclude children with albinism from group activities.

The cultural power of the melanocyte ranges from subtle variations of bias and insult to acts of extreme evil. Diseases such as vitiligo and albinism unfold in infinite variations, depending on the country and the players. We have used color to grade each other as superior or inferior, and made untold numbers of decisions based on skin color [1].

One of my own most vivid experiences with skin color occurred when I was a volunteer in Haiti and I stayed in the same building that housed an orphanage, medical clinic, and school. I remember walking up to the second floor to the orphanage and seeing the children that were left for adoption. In each of the cribs were infants–at least 5 or 6 in each crib. I remember lifting up several of the children and giving them hugs. I asked about the adoptions and the nurse told me that, "The light skin ones will be the only ones that will probably ever be adopted."

Tanzania is a nightmare for those with albinism. Because of bizarre beliefs by certain witch doctors, who far outnumber conventional doctors, those with albinism are in constant terror. More than 60 people have been killed in recent times by those hunting albinos for their legs, arms, hands and blood, which are put into potions to supposedly bring good luck and wealth. For those who survive, the horrendous acts of brutality have left many with double amputations of arms and legs, with limbs cut off and sold in Black Market trade. On a BBC report, it was noted that a witch doctor had offered $2000 for the arm of an albino.

Summary

Perhaps one day we will live in a world where color is am objective descriptor and not the defining or limiting character, echoed in the words of Martin Luther King, Jr.'s famous "I Have A Dream" speech, when he said, "I have a dream that my four little children will one day live in a nation where they will not be judged by the color of their skin but by the content of their character." Along the way, perhaps we can adapt more helpful scientific and cultural considerations to eliminate the bias of skin color. We hope in the future we will have genetic mechanisms, immunizations, and other ways to mend our skin ecosystem to prevent skin color abnormalities that make us prone to the rampant destruction of skin cancers, visual disturbances, and biochemical abnormalities. But for now, we must still struggle against the tragedy brought on by the craziness of distorted beliefs about skin color and character.

The melanocyte is part of the crucial structure at the bottom of the epidermis. The difference in concentration of its inherent melanin determines skin color and often determines the course of a person's life. The melanocyte—a tiny element of the skin–has been a key determinant of history and continues to drive much of what happens in the world of humans.

References

1. Norman R. The blue man and other stories of the skin. Oakland, California: University of California Press; 2014.
2. Jablonski N. Living color: the biological and social meaning of skin color. Oakland, California: University of California Press; 2014.

Chapter 11
Genome and Skin Cancer

Sharad P. Paul

Abstract The purpose of this chapter is to give an overview of skin cancer from a genomic perspective and provide an insight into new therapeutic targets as a result of these findings.

Keywords Genome • Skin cancer • Therapy

In my book, Skin, a Biography [1], I describe how skin and nerve cells develop at the same time, and the genetic signals that determine this differentiation. Investigators with The Cancer Genome Atlas (TCGA) Research Network have provided new insights into the genomic workings of deadly types of brain and skin cancers [2]. In one study, TCGA researchers from over 50 institutions and more than five countries analyzed the genomes of 333 melanoma skin tumors, identifying molecular subtypes that may help clinicians determine which tumors are more aggressive and which are more likely to respond to certain treatments [2]. Writing in *Cancer Cell*, these researchers report that cutaneous, or skin, melanomas can be grouped into one of four subtypes, which are based on genetic mutations: BRAF mutant, RAS mutant, NF1 mutant and Triple-WT (wild-type). Such genomic classification leads to individualized therapy for melanoma, the most aggressive and lethal skin cancer. For example, Triple-WT tumor subtype is characterized by mutations in growth-promoting enzymes called receptor tyrosine kinases, which could potentially be treated with drugs that inhibit their activity [3].

S.P. Paul, MD, MPhil
School of Medicine, University of Queensland, St Lucia, QLD, Australia

Director, Skin Surgery Clinic, Senior Lecturer, Faculty of Surgery, University of Auckland, Auckland, New Zealand

Adjunct Professor, Auckland University of Technology, Auckland, New Zealand
e-mail: sharad@sharadpaul.com

R.A. Norman (ed.), *Personalized, Evolutionary, and Ecological Dermatology*,
DOI 10.1007/978-3-319-41088-3_11

Firstly, melanoma rates are rising worldwide and until recently very few therapies were effective for advanced melanoma, leading investigators to look more closely down the genomic highway. Given fair-skinned people are more likely to develop melanoma, it is widely accepted that melanoma risk is modulated by skin pigmentation patterns, such as those linked to MC1R polymorphisms [4] and early exposure to ultraviolet (UV) light [5] – either natural (sunlight) or artificial (tanning beds). While we associate skin cancers with UV exposure, several other factors that contribute to the increased incidences are known and in specific situations become major determinants – these risk factors include, exposure to arsenic through drinking water, and organ-transplant associated immunosuppression [6]. Viral infections are also implicated in both non-melanoma skin cancers and more rare aggressive Merkel cell tumors – with various strains of human-papilloma viruses identified and increased incidences reported in individuals infected with HIV [7–10].

Given we now accept that there is no such thing as a safe tan, it is worth looking at the genetics of pigmentation and understand the many genes involved. The table below [11] summarizes the genes involved in the formation of the pigment, melanin. In this chapter, I will discuss the significance of each of these genes with respect to skin cancer, especially melanoma (see Table 11.1).

The MC1R gene is a major contributor to skin pigmentation. Figure 11.1 illustrates the synthesis of melanin. The gene consists of one single exon, and is highly polymorphic.

As illustrated in Fig. 11.1, low TYR activity will result in synthesis of yellow pheomelanin, which is responsible for the red hair and fair skin phenotype. The red hair and fair skin also represents the phenotype of individuals with truncated MC1R protein, which is also called as null genotype [12]. Studies have shown that MC1R variants are also associated with reduced apoptosis and inefficient DNA repair in melanocytes [13]. The link between the highly polymorphic MC1R gene and risk of BCC, SCC and melanoma has been consistently shown in several studies [14]. The R163Q variant, which is shown specifically to be associated with risk of BCC, results in a receptor with decreased surface expression and reduced affinity for a-MSH. However, as evidenced by the no effect of the MC1R variants in an Icelandic population, the frequency and nature of MC1R polymorphisms and effect on the risk of melanoma seems to vary between different populations [15]. Lastly, some studies

Table 11.1 Genes associated with common pigmentation traits

	Eye color	Hair color	Skin pigment/skin sensitivity
MCIR	–	+	+
ASIP	+	+	+
TYR	+	+	+
TYRP1	+	+	–
OCA2/HERC2	+	+	+
SLC24A4	+	+	+
KITLG	–	+	–
TPCN2	–	+	–
Chr 6 p25.3	–	+	+

Adapted from Scherer and Kumar [11]

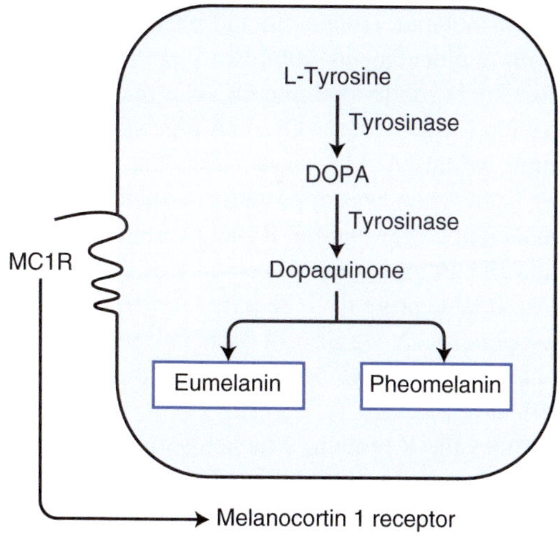

Fig. 11.1 Melanin synthesis and the role of TYR and MC1R (Adapted from Paul [1])

have also shown the association between germ line MC1R variants and frequency of somatic BRAF mutations in melanoma tumors with increased mutation frequency in patients with MC1R variants, while others studies have found no such link [16].

Agouti signaling protein (ASIP) was first described to inhibit eumelanogenesis in human melanocytes in 1997 [17]. In animals, this agouti gene has four different forms or alleles – the four alleles of agouti each produce a different pattern:

AS = makes solid color patterns

AY = produces a fawn or sable coat

AW = wild type — produces coats for wild animals like wolves

AT = produces black or tan coats

The ASIP gene is located on chromosome 20q and consists of three exons. A single nucleotide polymorphism in the 30UTR (rs6058017) of the ASIP gene, often designated as A8818G polymorphism, has been reported to be associated with dark hair and brown eyes in Caucasian populations [18]. When low ASIP protein levels are found, its inhibiting effect is diminished, while eumelanogenesis is increased, favoring dark pigmentation. When the rs6058017 variant is considered, decreased risk of BCC for carriers of the rs6058017, but not with SCC or melanoma is found [19]. A GWAS (genome-wide association study) reported the association of a haplotype which is located 100 kb upstream of the ASIP gene with pigmentation traits such as hair color, skin sensitivity to sun and freckling [20]. Another GWAS showed an association between polymorphisms downstream of ASIP and pigmentation traits as well as risk of cutaneous melanoma [21].

As illustrated in Fig. 11.1, Tyrosinase or TYR is a copper dependent enzyme that catalyzes the first two steps during melanogenesis. The protein is required for the synthesis of both types of melanin, eumelanin and pheomelanin. Mutations in the gene are associated with oculocutaneous albinism type 1 (OCA1), an autosomal recessive disorder. Albinism is subdivided into OCA1A and OCA1B depending on the severity of the disorder. Cases with the OCA1A type suffer from complete lifelong absence of melanin, while OCA1B cases retain the ability to tan [22]. The R402Q variant of the TYR gene was repeatedly associated with pigmentation traits – a significant association between the R402Q variant, and risk of cutaneous melanoma and of basal cell carcinoma was observed [23].

TYRP1 or Tyrosinase-related protein 1 is required for the synthesis of eumelanin but not for pheomelanogenesis. A significant association of the TYRP1 variant, rs1408799, and risk of melanoma has been found in three independent studies including a GWAS [19].

The OCA2 gene encodes the P protein, a melanosomal transmembrane protein that is involved in small molecule transport into melanosomes, thus triggering melanogenesis. Mutations in the gene cause the most common form of oculocutaneous albinism, OCA2, wherein the gene derives its name from. Two studies revealed a significantly-increased risk of cutaneous melanoma for carriers of the OCA2 R419Q variant (rs1800407). However, this could not be confirmed in a study on female nurses [15]. Interestingly, a study based on a French population showed significant association of OCA2 variants with risk of melanoma [19].

When we consider the solute carrier families (SLC), SLC24A4 and SLC24A5 are potassium-dependent sodium/calcium exchangers, bound to the melanosomal membrane. The SLC24A5 gene influenced skin color development by breeding out the environmentally incompatible African skin type in European conditions, when man first ventured out of Africa [24]. Another solute carrier gene, SLC24A4, determines green eyes rather than blue eyes [25]. However, both these solute carriers have not been associated with BCC or melanoma.

The Kit ligand, KITLG binds to the tyrosine receptor kinase KIT and consequently promotes migration, survival and proliferation of melanocytes. It is now known that humans with two copies of the African form of the KITLG gene have darker skin color, when compared to people with one or two copies of the new KITLG variant that is common in Europe. Interestingly, lightly-colored fish also have regulatory mutations that reduce expression of the KITLG gene in gills and skin – Sticklebacks changed skin color to adapt to freshwater colors and camouflage themselves; humans changed skin color based on the need for sun protection [26]. However, variants of KITLG also did not show an association with melanoma or with BCC [15].

Two-pore segment channel 2 (TPCN2) and IRF4/Chr6: The investigation of these variants for their effect on skin cancer showed no significant association with either BCC or cutaneous melanoma [15].

Thus, the phenotype alone is not sufficient to predict a person's risk of skin cancer. It is however felt that the MC1R genotype might affect the histology of nevi and melanomas [27]. A recent study also showed a significant association between MC1R genotype and sensitivity to psoralen-ultraviolet A (PUVA) phototherapy (Fig. 11.2) [29].

Interestingly, when one studies genetic alterations in melanomas, melanomas from skin with evidence of chronic sun damage, intermittent sun exposure without

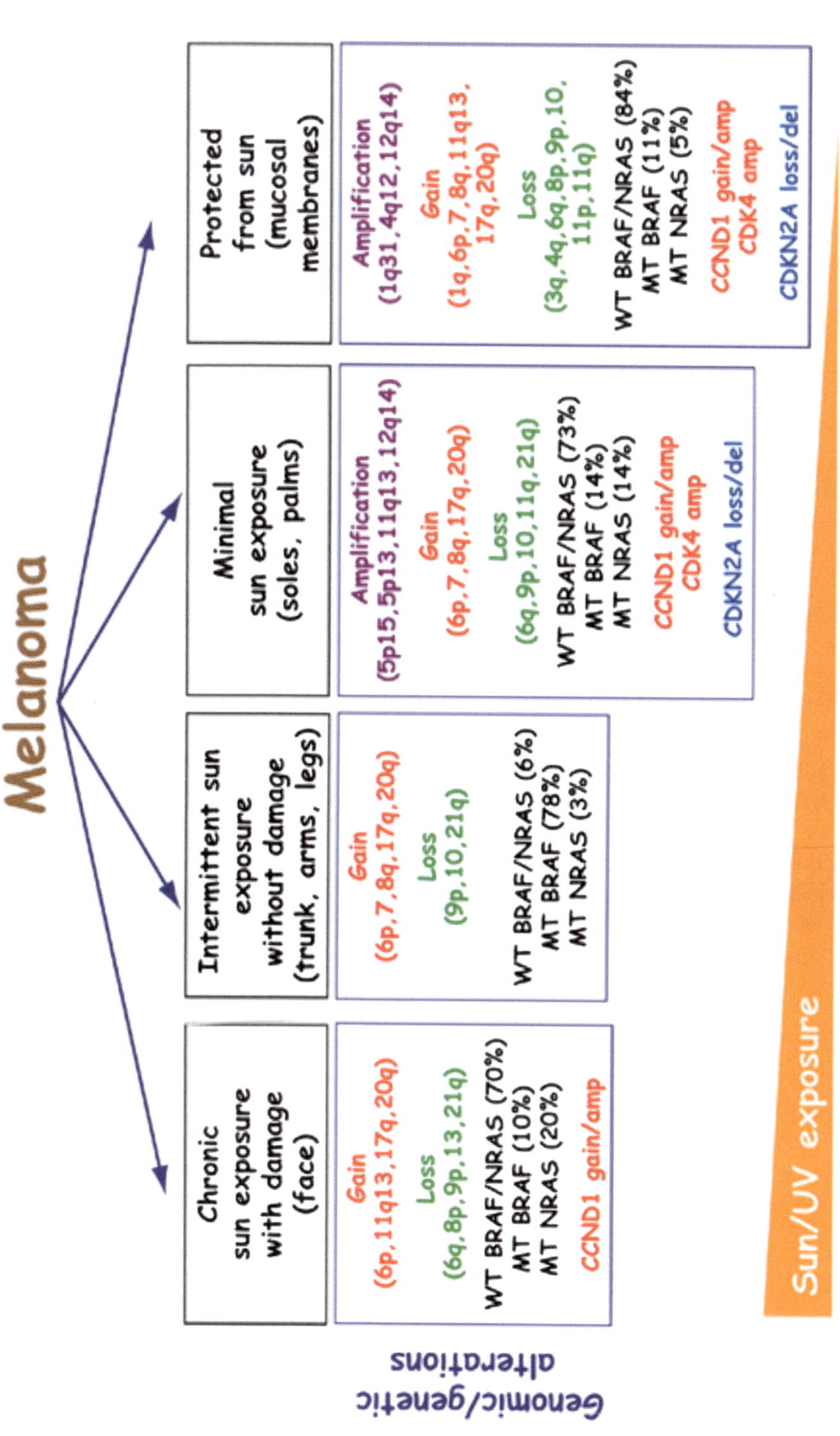

Fig. 11.2 Summary of genetic alterations in melanomas from patients with varying degrees of sun exposure as reported by Curtin et al. [31] (Adapted from Kabbarah and Chin [3])

evidence of damage, and no significant exposure exhibit distinct genomic patterns of gain/amplification and loss/deletion and different BRAF/NRAS mutational spectrums. BRAF and NRAS mutations were mutually exclusive, as were BRAF/NRAS activating mutations and increased copies of CCND1 or CDK4. Gain/amplification of CDK4 was more commonly seen in melanomas from protected skin than in melanoma from sun-exposed skin, as was deletion/loss of the CDNK2A locus, which was observed exclusively in samples without CDK4 amplification. UV, ultraviolet light; WT, wildtype; MT, mutant; amp, amplification [3].

The recognition of the genomic heterogeneity of different types of melanoma has important clinical and therapeutic implications, as it has a direct impact on design of clinical studies and therapeutic approaches. For example, since activation of MAPK (BRAF/NRAS) and the PI3K pathways are important in the subgroup of melanoma from skin with intermittent UV exposure, which is the most common form of the disease, BRAF may provide a logical target for therapeutic intervention [30]. Conversely, in the case of melanomas from chronically sun-damaged skin or from UV-protected sites, which typically do not acquire BRAF mutations but rather amass higher copy numbers of CCND1 or CDK4, a therapeutic approach involving CDK inhibitors might yield a positive response and this is something researchers are actively pursuing [31].

Let's look at the genetics of basal cell cancers, which are the skin commonest cancers. The discovery of mutations in the patched 1 (PTCH1) gene in the germ line of people with Gorlin syndrome (also known as nevoid basal cell carcinoma syndrome) and in sporadic BCC led to the identification of the importance of the HH signaling pathway in human carcinogenesis, Indeed, PTCH1 is part of the hedgehog signaling pathway, and derangements within this pathway are now known to be important in the carcinogenesis of many different cancers including sporadic basal cell carcinoma [28].

Gorlin syndrome, described above was first described in 1960 [32] and is a rare autosomal dominant disorder characterized by three major features: multiple BCC, dyskeratotic palmar and plantar pitting, and odontogenic keratocysts. People with this syndrome are born with an inherited mutation of one allele of the PTCH1 gene, the majority of which lead to truncation of the PTCH1 protein, thus representing a null allele [33].

The HH signaling pathway is involved in the regulation of growth and patterning in embryos, and has also been implicated in the maintenance of stem or progenitor cells in many adult tissues, consistent with its involvement in human carcinogenesis [34]. PTCH1 is part of a receptor complex at the cell surface made up of two transmembrane proteins PTCH1 and smoothened (SMO) [35]. Hedgehog is a secreted protein that binds to PTCH1 to activate the pathway. The hedgehog interacting protein (HIP) binds to HH and acts as a negative regulator of the pathway. In the excellent review article on the genetics of BCC, Zwaan and others have illustrated this pathway very well (Fig. 11.3) [36]. The same Gorlin syndrome PTCH1 gene mutation is seen in up to 70 % of sporadic BCC in people without Gorlin syndrome [37].

The gene P53 encodes the protein P53 which has been termed 'guardian of the genome' – given disruption of this pathway occurs in most human tumours [38]. A germ line mutation in P53 causes a cancer predisposition syndrome called Li-Fraumeni syndrome [39]. Basal cell carcinoma is not predisposed to by this

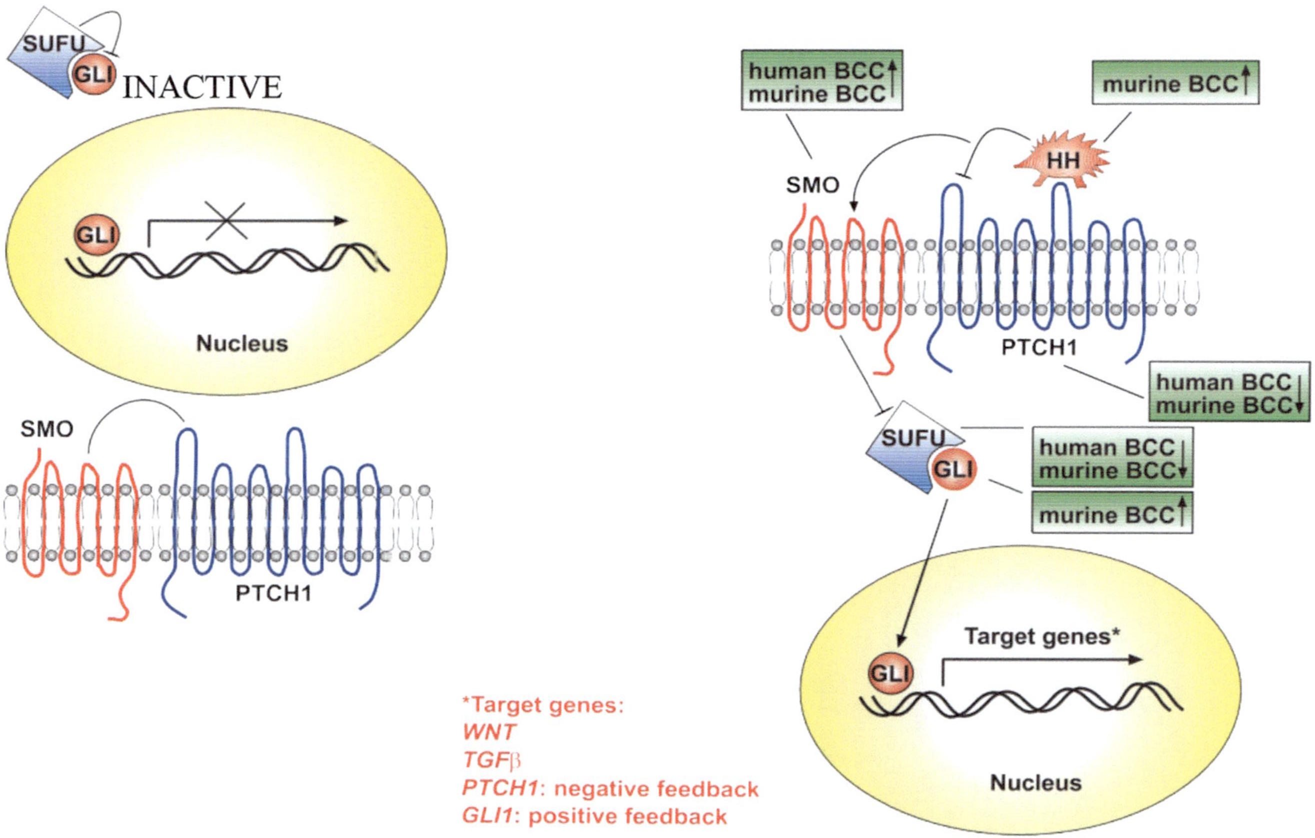

Fig. 11.3 Simplified image of the inactive and active hedgehog (HH) signaling pathways, and alterations in BCC. Active patched 1 (PTCH1) inhibits smoothened (SMO) and results in the inactivation of the HH signaling pathway (Adapted from de Zwaan and Haass [36])

syndrome, suggesting that P53 mutation is not necessary for BCC genesis, but instead may be a secondary event. This is confirmed by studies in sunscreen users – people using sunscreen had significantly less P53 mutations in their BCC compared with those not using sunscreen, also suggesting that P53 mutation is a secondary event and not required for BCC carcinogenesis [40]. The P53-regulated gene 14-3-3 s has reduced or absent protein expression in BCC. The protein encoded by this gene is essential for senescence of keratinocytes and thus loss of the gene may contribute to growth of keratinizing tumours [41]. In other keratinizing tumors such as SCC, a recent report highlighted the discovery of recurrent mutations concentrated at an ultraviolet signature hotspot in KNSTRN, which encodes a kinetochore protein, in 19 % of cutaneous squamous cell carcinomas (SCC). Cancer-associated KNSTRN mutations, most notably those encoding p. Ser24Phe, disrupt chromatid cohesion in normal cells, occur in SCC precursors, correlate with increased aneuploidy in primary tumors and enhance tumorigenesis in vivo. These findings suggest a role for KNSTRN mutagenesis in SCC development [42]. Looking at keratinocytes, Mouse models of BCC carcinogenesis suggest that dysregulation of the HH pathway is essential for development of BCC: In transgenic mice, BCC or BCC-like tumors were generated by overexpression of Hh, Gli1, Gli2 or activating mutation of Smo or by heterozygous Ptch± or Sufu± in keratinocytes [43].

We have earlier looked at pigmentation-related genes implicated in BCC and melanoma. There are some other genes that could also possibly be significant in skin cancers:

Human papillomavirus: More than 100 subtypes of HPV have been identified and are divided into the phylogenetic genera a, b, g, m and n. Whereas b-HPV are associated with SCC in immunocompromized and immunocompetent people and those with epidermodysplasia verruciformis, they are not yet consistently identified in BCC [44].

Glutathione-S-transferases: Associations with BCC have been seen in immunosuppressed people, those with Gorlin syndrome, people with multiple BCC, and in the general population although no single glutathione-S-transferase or CYP enzyme gene has consistently shown to affect risk [45].

Cyclin-dependent kinase inhibitor 2A – P16INK4A and P14ARF: The cyclin-dependent kinase inhibitor 2A (CDKN2A) locus is mutated in many human cancers including malignant melanoma. It encodes two proteins with cell cycle regulatory roles: P16INK4A and P14ARF. However, very recently a variant at 9q21 (containing both CDKN2A and CDKN2B genes) was noted as a predisposition locus for BCC, but not melanoma [46].

Keratin 5: Variants of the basal keratinocyte keratin K5 (the heteromeric partner of K14) – especially the G138E variant – affects BCC susceptibility independently from risk for cutaneous melanoma or any pigmentation trait [46].

Brahma: A genetic analysis of Brahma (BRM) in human NMSC, precancerous lesions and normal skin revealed a common point mutation present in one of 10 SCC and two of six BCC – reflecting UVA damage where A:T to G:C transversion and dimer formation occurs. This 'hotspot mutation' occurs in a highly conserved region of the BRM gene [47].

Gap junctions: These are typically made up of connexins – Cx26 is induced, and Cx43 decreased in BCC [48]; Cx43 is present in the cytoplasm and in poorly developed gap junctions in both BCC and SCC [49].

Targeting Treatment

Therapies involving inhibition of Hedgehog (HH) signaling are expected to suppress tumor growth of BCC based on research results. A steroidal alkaloid of the lily Veratrum californicum, cyclopamine, inhibits HH signaling and reverses the effects of oncogenic SMO and PTCH1 mutations and has shown some promise [50]. The retinoid tazarotene has recently shown promise as a topical chemopreventive agent against BCC, again by down-regulating the HH pathway [51]. In January 2012, vismodegib (Erivedge; Curis/Genentech), a small-molecule inhibitor of the Hedgehog signaling pathway, was approved by the US Food and Drug Administration (FDA) for the treatment of basal cell carcinoma (BCC) [52].

Although genetic factors have been identified for melanoma as discussed earlier, only 10 % or less of all melanoma cases arise in families with clusters of melanoma [53].

Nearly 40 % of families with at least 3 melanoma cases demonstrated mutations in the major hereditary melanoma susceptibility gene, CDKN2A; however, more than 50 % of such high-risk families demonstrate no known genetic mutation [54]. A summary of the genes under investigation for melanoma is found in the table below (Table 11.2) [56].

The table above lists the germline and somatic mutations in melanoma. Of these, only BRAF and CDKN2A have been identified as realistic therapeutic targets thus far.

BRAF regulation of melanoma cell survival has emerged as a target for therapy. The BRAF kinase inhibitor vemurafenib demonstrated improved overall and progression-free survival in stage IIIC and IV melanoma [57]. Accordingly, the US Food and Drug Administration (FDA) granted approval in 2011 for the use of vemurafenib in patients with BRAF V600E mutated unresectable metastatic melanoma; FDA in 2014 granted approval for the use of dabrafenib in the treatment of BRAF V600E mutated unresectable metastatic melanoma [58].

Greater Breslow thickness in cutaneous melanoma is also found to correlate with the presence of a CDKN2A mutation. Patients with the CDKN2A mutation also had increased risks of pancreatic, breast, gastrointestinal, and lung cancers and Wilms tumor, suggesting additional genetic modifiers [59]. It has also been shown that CDKN2A mutation carriers who develop melanoma do so at a younger age than patients with CDKN2A wild-type melanoma, at a median age of 39 versus 54.3 years [60]. CDKN2A has been widely studied as a candidate gene for melanoma – however, these results have not been validated sufficiently to translate into a specific genetic test that assesses the risk of developing these phenotypes in the general population [55].

Table 11.2 Germline and somatic mutations seen in melanoma

Gene	Location	Function	Application in melanoma
N-RAS	1p13-p11 Somatic mutation	Encodes NRAS, cell cycle regulation	Under investigation
H-RAS	11p15.5 Somatic mutation	Encodes HRAS, transforming protein p21, cell cycle regulation	Under investigation
BRAF	**7q34** **Somatic mutation**	**Encodes BRAF, cell cycle regulation**	**Selection of patients for targeted therapy**
CDKN2A	**9p21.3** **Germline mutation**	**Encodes CDKN2A, p16, p14ARF, cell cycle regulation**	**Selection of patients for closer screening and surveillance**
TERT	10p15 Germline and somatic mutations	Encodes hTERT, regulation of telomerase and cellular senescence	Under investigation
POT1	7q31.33 Germline mutation	Encodes POT1, regulation of telomerase and cellular senescence	Under investigation
CDK4	12q14.1 Germline and somatic mutations	Encodes CDK4, cell cycle regulation	Under investigation
BAP1	3p12.31-p21.2 Germline and somatic mutations	Encodes BAP1, regulates DNA repair	Under investigation
PTEN	10q23.31 Germline mutation	Encodes PTEN, cell cycle regulation	Under investigation
MC1R	16q24.3 Somatic mutation	Encodes MC1R, encodes skin and hair pigment	Under investigation
MITF	3p14-p13 Germline and somatic mutations	Encodes MITF, regulates melanocyte development	Under investigation
BRCA2	13q12.3 Germline mutation	Encodes BRCA2, regulates DNA repair	Under investigation

Adapted from Zager and Rashid [55]

References

1. Paul SP. Skin, a biography. 4th ed. 2013.
2. Benowitz S. Peering at brain and skin cancers through a genomic lens, scientists begin to rewrite rules for identifying tumor types. National Human Genome Research Institute. https://www.genome.gov/27561001. Accessed 8 Oct 2015.
3. Kabbarah O, Chin L. Revealing the genomic heterogeneity of melanoma. Cancer Cell. 2005;8(6):439–41.
4. Palmer JS, Duffy DL, et al. Melanocortin-1 receptor polymorphisms and risk of melanoma: is the association explained solely by pigmentation phenotype? Am J Hum Genet. 2000;66:176–86.
5. Thompson JF, Scolyer RA, Kefford RF. Cutaneous melanoma. Lancet. 2005;365:687–701.

6. Ahsan H, Chen Y, Kibriya MG, Slavkovich V, Parvez F, Jasmine F, Gamble MV, Graziano JH. Arsenic metabolism, genetic susceptibility, and risk of premalignant skin lesions in Bangladesh. Cancer Epidemiol Biomarkers Prev. 2007;16:1270–8.
7. Guo X, Fujino Y, Ye X, Liu J, Yoshimura T. Association between multi-level inorganic arsenic exposure from drinking water and skin lesions in China. Int J Environ Res Public Health. 2006;3:262–7.
8. Euvrard S, Kanitakis J, Claudy A. Skin cancers after organ transplantation. N Engl J Med. 2003;348:1681–91.
9. Engels EA. Non-AIDS-defining malignancies in HIV-infected persons: etiologic puzzles, epidemiologic perils, prevention opportunities. AIDS. 2009;23:875–85.
10. Feng H, Shuda M, Chang Y, Moore PS. Clonal integration of a polyomavirus in human Merkel cell carcinoma. Science. 2008;319:1096–100.
11. Scherer R, Kumar R. Genetics of pigmentation in skin cancer—a review. Mutat Res. 2010;705:141–53.
12. Beaumont KA, Shekar SN, et al. Red hair is the null phenotype of MC1R. Hum Mutat. 2008;29(8):E88–94.
13. Bohm M, Wolff I, Scholzen TE, Robinson SJ, Healy E, Luger TA, Schwarz T, Schwarz A. alpha-Melanocyte-stimulating hormone protects from ultraviolet radiation-induced apoptosis and DNA damage. J Biol Chem. 2005;280:5795–802.
14. Han J, Kraft P, et al. A genome-wide association study identifies novel alleles associated with hair color and skin pigmentation. PLoS Genet. 2008;4:e1000074.
15. Gudbjartsson DF, Sulem P, Stacey SN, Goldstein AM, et al. ASIP and TYR pigmentation variants associate with cutaneous melanoma and basal cell carcinoma. Nat Genet. 2008;40:886–91.
16. Landi MT, Bauer J, Pfeiffer RM, et al. MC1R germline variants confer risk for BRAF- mutant melanoma. Science. 2006;313:521–2.
17. Suzuki I, Tada A, Ollmann MM, et al. Agouti signaling protein inhibits melanogenesis and the response of human melanocytes to alpha-melanotropin. J Invest Dermatol. 1997;108:838–42.
18. Norton HL, Kittles RA, Parra E, McKeigue P, et al. Genetic evidence for the convergent evolution of light skin in Europeans and East Asians. Mol Biol Evol. 2007;24:710–22.
19. Nan H, Kraft P, Hunter DJ, Han J. Genetic variants in pigmentation genes, pigmentary phenotypes, and risk of skin cancer in Caucasians. Int J Cancer. 2009;129:2250–7.
20. Sulem P, Gudbjartsson DF, Stacey SN, et al. Two newly identified genetic determinants of pigmentation in Europeans. Nat Genet. 2008;40:835–7.
21. Brown KM, Macgregor S, Montgomery GW, et al. Common sequence variants on 20q11.22 confer melanoma susceptibility. Nat Genet. 2008;40:838–40.
22. Oetting WS. The tyrosinase gene and oculocutaneous albinism type 1 (OCA1): a model for understanding the molecular biology of melanin formation. Pigment Cell Res. 2000,113:320–5.
23. Duffy DL, Zhao ZZ, Sturm RA, Hayward NK, et al. Multiple pigmentation gene polymorphisms account for a substantial propor-tion of risk of cutaneous malignant melanoma. J Invest Dermatol. 2010;130:520–8.
24. Paul SP. Skin, a biography. 4th ed. 2013. p. 119.
25. Paul SP. Skin, a biography. 4th ed. 2013. p. 124.
26. Paul SP. Skin, a biography. 4th ed. 2013. p. 80.
27. Zalaudek I, Meiklejohn W, Argenziano G, Thurber AE, Sturm RA. “White” nevi and “red” melanomas: association with the RHC phenotype of the MC1R gene. Invest Dermatol. 2009;129:1305.
28. Hahn H, Wicking C, Zaphiropoulous PG, et al. Mutations of the human homolog of Drosophila patched in the nevoid basal cell carcinoma syndrome. Cell. 1996;85:841–51.
29. Smith G, Wilkie MJ, Deeni YY, Farr PM, Ferguson J, Wolf CR, Ibbotson SH. Melanocortin 1 receptor (MC1R) genotype influences erythemal sensitivity to psoralen-ultraviolet A photochemotherapy. Br J Dermatol. 2007;157:1230–4.

30. Tuveson DA, Weber BL, Herlyn M. BRAF as a potential therapeutic target in melanoma and other malignancies. Cancer Cell. 2003;4:95–8.
31. Curtin JA, Fridlyand J, Kageshita T, et al. Distinct sets of genetic alterations in melanoma. N Engl J Med. 2005;353(20):2135–47.
32. Gorlin RJ, Goltz RW. Multiple nevoid basal-cell epithelioma, jaw cysts and bifid rib. A syndrome. N Engl J Med. 1960;262:908–12.
33. Wicking C, Shanley S, Smyth I, et al. Most germ-line mutations in the nevoid basal cell carcinoma syndrome lead to a premature termination of the PATCHED protein, and no genotype-phenotype correlations are evident. Am J Hum Genet. 1997;60:21–6.
34. Jiang J, Hui CC. Hedgehog signaling in development and cancer. Dev Cell. 2008;15:801–12.
35. Stone DM, Hynes M, Armanini M, et al. The tumor-suppressor gene patched encodes a candidate receptor for Sonic hedgehog. Nature. 1996;384:129–34.
36. De Zwaan SE, Haass NK. Genetics of basal cell carcinoma: review. Aust J Dermatol. 2010;51:81–94.
37. Aszterbaum M, Rothman A, Johnson RL, et al. Identification of mutations in the human PATCHED gene in sporadic basal cell carcinomas and in patients with the basal cell nevus syndrome. J Invest Dermatol. 1998;110:885–8.
38. Lane DP. Cancer. p53, 'guardian of the genome.'. Nature. 1992;358:15–6.
39. Malkin D, Li FP, Strong LC, et al. Germ line p53 mutations in a familial syndrome of breast cancer, sarcomas, and other neoplasms. Science. 1990;250:1233–8.
40. Rosenstein BS, Phelps RG, Weinstock MA, et al. p53 mutations in basal cell carcinomas arising in routine users of sunscreens. Photochem Photobiol. 1999;70:798–806.
41. Lodygin D, Yazdi AS, Sander CA, et al. Analysis of 14-3-3sigma expression in hyperproliferative skin diseases reveals selective loss associated with CpG-methylation in basal cell carcinoma. Oncogene. 2003;22:5519–24.
42. Lee CS, Bhaduri A, Khavari P, et al. Recurrent point mutations in the kinetochore gene KNSTRN in cutaneous squamous cell carcinoma. Nat Genet. 2014;46:1060–2.
43. Svard J, Rozell B, Toftgard R, et al. Tumor suppressor gene co-operativity in compound Patched1 and suppressor of fused heterozygous mutant mice. Mol Carcinog. 2008;9:9.
44. Karagas MR, Nelson HH, She P, et al. Human papillomavirus infection and incidence of squamous cell and basal cell carcinomas of the skin. J Natl Cancer Inst. 2006;98:389–95.
45. Yang XR, Pfeiffer RM, Goldstein AM. Influence of glutathione-S-transferase (GSTM1, GSTP1, GSTT1) and cytochrome p450 (CYP1A1, CYP2D6) polymorphisms on numbers of basal cell carcinomas (BCCs) in families with the naevoid basal cell carcinoma syndrome. J Med Genet. 2006;43:e16.
46. Stacey SN, Sulem P, Masson G, et al. New common variants affecting susceptibility to basal cell carcinoma. Nat Genet. 2009;41:909–14.
47. Moloney FJ, Lyons JG, Bock VL, et al. Hotspot mutation of Brahma in non-melanoma skin cancer. J Invest Dermatol. 2009;129:1012–5.
48. Wilgenbus KK, Kirkpatrick CJ, Knuechel R, et al. Expression of Cx26, Cx32 and Cx43 gap junction proteins in normal and neoplastic human tissues. Int J Cancer. 1992;51:522–9.
49. Tada J, Hashimoto K. Ultrastructural localization of gap junction protein connexin 43 in normal human skin, basal cell carcinoma, and squamous cell carcinoma. J Cutan Pathol. 1997;24:628–35.
50. Taipale J, Chen JK, Cooper MK, et al. Effects of oncogenic mutations in Smoothened and Patched can be reversed by cyclopamine. Nature. 2000;406:1005–9.
51. So PL, Fujimoto MA, Epstein Jr EH. Pharmacologic retinoid signaling and physiologic retinoic acid receptor signaling inhibit basal cell carcinoma tumorigenesis. Mol Cancer Ther. 2008;7:1275–84.
52. Dlugosz A, Agrawal S, Kirkpatrick P. Vismodegib. Nat Rev Drug Discov. 2012;11:437–8.
53. Berwick M, Orlow L, Hummer AJ, et al. The prevalence of CDKN2A germ-line mutations and relative risk for cutaneous malignant melanoma: an international population-based study. Cancer Epidemiol Biomarkers Prev. 2006;15:1520–5.

54. Goldstein AM, Chan M, Harland M, et al. High-risk melanoma susceptibility genes and pancreatic cancer, neural system tumors, and uveal melanoma across *GenoMEL*. Cancer Res. 2006;66:9818–28.
55. Zager OM, Rashid JM. Genetic testing in the multidisciplinary management of melanoma. Surg Oncol Clin N Am. 2015;24(4):779–93.
56. Rashid JM. Genetic testing in the multidisciplinary management of melanoma. Surg Oncol Clin N Am. 2015;24(4):779–93.
57. Chapman PB, Hauschild A, Robert C, et al. Improved survival with vemurafenib in melanoma with BRAF V600E mutation. N Engl J Med. 2011;364:2507–16.
58. Hauschild A, Grob JJ, Demidov LV, et al. Dabrafenib in BRAF-mutated metastatic melanoma: a multicentre, open-label, phase 3 randomised controlled trial. Lancet. 2012;380:358–65.
59. Mukherjee B, Delancey JO, Raskin L, et al. Risk of non-melanoma cancers in first-degree relatives of CDKN2A mutation carriers. J Natl Cancer Inst. 2012;104:953–6.
60. van der Rhee JI, Krijnen P, Gruis NA, et al. Clinical and histologic characteristics of malignant melanoma in families with a germline mutation in CDKN2A. J Am Acad Dermatol. 2011;65:281–8.

Index

R.A. Norman (ed.), *Personalized, Evolutionary, and Ecological Dermatology*,
DOI 10.1007/978-3-319-41088-3

MIX
Papier aus verantwortungsvollen Quellen
Paper from responsible sources
FSC® C105338

If you have any concerns about our products,
you can contact us on
ProductSafety@springernature.com

In case Publisher is established outside the EU,
the EU authorized representative is:
Springer Nature Customer Service Center GmbH
Europaplatz 3, 69115 Heidelberg, Germany

Printed by Libri Plureos GmbH
in Hamburg, Germany